A time to
LOVE

A time to
LOVE

HELEN M. HOSTETLER

HERALD PRESS
Scottdale, Pennsylvania
Kitchener, Ontario

Library of Congress Cataloging-in-Publication Data
Hostetler, Helen M., 1922-
　A time to love / Helen M. Hostetler.
　　p.　cm.
　ISBN 0-8361-3504-0 (alk. paper)
　1. Hostetler, Roger—Health.　2. AIDS (Disease)—Patients—
California—Biography.　3. Christian life—1960-　I. Title.
RC607.A26H67　1989
362.1'969792'0092—dc20
[B]　　　　　　　　　　　　　　　　　　　　　　　89-33683
　　　　　　　　　　　　　　　　　　　　　　　　　　　CIP

A TIME TO LOVE
Copyright © 1989 by Herald Press, Scottdale, Pa. 15683
　Published simultaneously in Canada by Herald Press,
　Kitchener, Ont. N2G 4M5. All rights reserved.
Library of Congress Catalog Card Number: 89-33683
International Standard Book Number: 0-8361-3504-0
Printed in the United States of America
Cover art by Gwen Stamm
Design by Paula M. Johnson

95 94 93 92 91 90 89 10 9 8 7 6 5 4 3 2 1

To Roger
Our beloved son
Who
Through pain and struggle
For identity, acceptance, and love,
Gave up life, but found eternal peace.
We loved you.

There is no fear in love. But perfect love drives out fear, because fear has to do with punishment. The one who fears is not made perfect in love. We love because he first loved us. If anyone says, "I love God," yet hates his brother, he is a liar. For anyone who does not love his brother, whom he has seen, cannot love God, whom he has not seen. And he has given us this command: Whoever loves God must also love his brother.

1 John 4:18-21

Contents

Acknowledgments and Thanks 9
Author's Preface 11

1. News from the West 15
2. A Grave Error 26
3. The Prophecy 34
4. A Dark Day in August 38
5. Unwelcome Guests 45
6. Love Made Visible 53
7. The Greatest of These Is Love 59
8. Reflections 63
9. AIDS Confirmed 77
10. Faithful Friends 82
11. Christmas 93
12. Last Will and Testament 102
13. A Plan for Transition 111
14. A Night of Celebration 119
15. One Last Wish 124
16. Time to Be Tender 130
17. Our Times Are in God's Hands 137
18. Missing Person 142
19. A Call for Help 144
20. The Chill of Chains 149
21. Courage in Times of Testing 157
22. Anxious Waiting 164
23. The Healing Team 170
24. A Day to Remember 179

25. Stretcher Bearers 184
26. The Last Farewell 190
27. Time for Tribute 196
28. Blessed Be Sorrow 209
29. Epilogue: A Time to Love 215

The Author 220

Acknowledgments and Thanks

1. To Esther Loewen Vogt, I wish to express my heartfelt appreciation for her helpful assistance in editing my original manuscript. Her affirmation and encouragement put fresh energy into completing our story.

2. To my dear husband, Marvin, who shared this journey with me; gave love, comfort, and encouragement and allowed me the time to write our story.

3. To our daughters and husbands, Sheryl and Leo Miller, and Janene and Bob Stockamp, who selflessly gave us continued support and love. They sacrificed of their time and finances to assist us. We could not have made it without their help.

4. To our pastor, Ed R. Stucky, and friends at First Mennonite Church, of McPherson, Kansas, who prayed with us, cried with us, and assisted us with gifts, notes of encouragement, and care.

5. To our friends at First Mennonite Fellowship at San Francisco, especially Pastor Ruth Buxman, for the gift of

love, her insight, prayers, and willingness to give hours of time and energy in assisting Roger in his quest for peace and forgiveness.

6. To Doug Basinger for the hours of physical and emotional energy invested in dealing with Roger's business affairs, assisting in his relocation, and acting as his power of attorney. For the encouragement that he and John gave us and the helpful assistance in liquidating all of Roger's personal belongings. We love you.

7. To Hospice of San Francisco for the many hours of professional and volunteer services provided for Roger's care. We are deeply grateful. You are very special to us.

8. To Shanti, which provided a residence for care and volunteers who became such a very important part of Roger's final days. For the love and care that you shared, we will be eternally grateful. You have demonstrated genuine love. You remain forever friends.

9. To all our friends and family, near and far, who have given support, prayed for Roger and us, and have given me encouragement to write our story, thank you. You have walked beside us in our pain and in our joys. May God bless you all.

Author's Preface

As parents who have given up a son to the deadly disease of AIDS, we have gained some maturity and insight into the complexities of life. Some meaning has been put into our questioning. In the mystery of pain and misunderstanding has come opportunity for learning and growth. We have been touched with God's healing power and have gained the strength to walk beside those who are suffering.

We value the risks that we took in being open and honest and allowing others to walk beside us to help bear our burdens. To encourage others, we share this story of pain through the long days and nights of dealing with the theological questions with our apparent failure in communicating faith as we understood it and with the deep hurt in seeing a loved one suffer so incredibly. The stigma expressed by Christians makes it difficult for persons with AIDS (acquired immune deficiency syndrome) to seek counsel and care from the Christian community. It is well to remember the words of admonition, "since *all* have sinned and fall short of the glory of God" (Romans 3:23; emphasis mine).

I encourage you to be a healing influence to your families, friends, and to the world. It was through the caring arms of God's children that we were sustained.

This book is not an attempt to deal with the homosexuality issue or an interpretation of the theological questions. It is simply a candid account of our personal journey, which has so drastically affected us and those we have come to love.

It is my hope that you too might gain some new understandings as we allow you to see into our very souls and observe the struggles, the questions, the pain, and also the triumphs, the hope, and the peace that evolved from surrendering to God. We trust that our story is a tribute to our dear son, Roger, whom we loved so much.

Helen M. Hostetler
McPherson, Kansas

A time to
LOVE

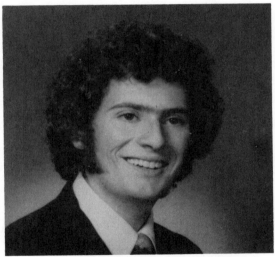

Roger Oliver Hostetler upon his graduation
from Goshen College in 1972 at age 22

1

News from the West

It was a mild February day of 1978 in south central Kansas. Thin, pale sunshine seeped from the sky and touched the crisp winter day with opaque light. I had the day off from my regular duties as a staff nurse at our local Memorial Hospital. Trying to cram a week's work into one day was the usual agenda, and one by one I scratched jobs off my "to do" list for the day.

As I paused to examine the refrigerator for a quick lunch idea, I saw through my kitchen window our faithful mail carrier slow to a stop at our mailbox. I hurriedly started lunch, went eagerly to the mailbox, and found a letter from our son Roger, now living in Felton, a suburb of San José, California. A letter from him was always welcome and I tore it open and began to read. The silk-screen printing business was booming, he said, and present quarters were too small, so they were moving to a larger space. He had just started a new 10-week EST training seminar on the body. He had lost fifteen pounds and was feeling trim and better about himself than he ever had and was anxious to get in touch with his body and physical capabilities. He was beginning an exercise routine in an effort to become more fit.

The letter continued:

Something I've wanted to share with you for a long time has been coming up a lot for me lately, and I've decided to put myself out there and let you know another part of me. That is—I'm gay. The first thing I want you to know is that it is *only* out of my experience of your absolute love for me that I can share this with you.

My mouth felt dry, my heart was racing, I could feel the pulse in my throat, and I thought I was going to choke. The words *I'm gay . . . I'm gay . . . I'm gay* seemed a part of my heartbeat. Tears filled my eyes, but I had to read on.

I've had nightmares about the process of letting you know . . . your response . . . and the effect it may have on our relationship. What I've gotten lately is that it needn't have any effect on our relationship and that our love for each other underlies any difference in attitudes and beliefs around sexual preference, and I know that is so and it gives me the space to share some of myself with you. It *is* who I am. I of course tried to deny it for ages, and after the denial period, years passed before I could bring myself to share it with another person. It has been a slow but steady process in coming to the place where I am now in accepting the fact that I am a homosexual. I've found that the more I share with people as to who I am, withholding nothing, the more support I receive in really *being* who I am.

For a long time I didn't think it necessary to tell you because . . . it must be a hard one for you and I didn't want to bring you additional grief. However, I don't feel like I can act out any more games in terms of my sexuality, with anyone. It's important for me that you know about my sexuality, because I've felt your wishes that I find the right girl . . . marriage . . . kids . . . and all. And, of course, it is not even a remote possibility and now I don't have to act like it is.

I also want you to know that I accept full responsibility for my life and who I am. Please don't try to figure out where you went wrong and all of that.

I'm completely satisfied and happy as I turned out and there is absolutely nothing for you to feel guilty about. I know it must be strange for you to be reading this. Again, I want to acknowledge you for loving me over and over until I finally got to a place in my life where I could experience that love as genuine, and giving me the space to tell you all of this.

I know that this is probably the hardest thing I've asked you to accept about me. And, I guess that's where I'm at. It doesn't matter if you accept that about me or not. As I said before, I know there is love for me from you which underlies things about me such as my lifestyle. It is from this place that I really want to relate to you rather than trying to come from our differences.

I have a relationship with a really wonderful man named _____ who lives in San Francisco. It is nurturing and supporting and by far the most natural and satisfying romantic relationship I've ever had. He turns out to be from Hutchinson. Small world. Anyway, he is a community organizer in the Tenderloin (the Bowery of San Francisco) and directs a writers' workshop in poetry in a program of resocialization through the arts. He is a powerful person involved in really challenging work, . . . an exciting person to relate to and grow with. He usually comes down on weekends as he likes the country more than I like the city.

I'm happy and I want you to know that.

Well, I don't know what else to say, so I guess I'll close and thank you for taking this all in.

I love you,
Roger

I stared through my kitchen window toward the stately oak trees framed by white billowy clouds and the wide, blue Kansas sky. Everything became one big blur as I looked through my tears. Sobs wrenched through my body as in agony I turned to the Lord, my source of comfort and strength. "O Lord, when I am overwhelmed, lead me to the Rock that is higher than I. You are my help and my deliverer, O Lord, do not delay. Be my rock of Refuge to which I can always go. You are my rock and my fortress" (see Psalms 61:2; 71:3).

In my jumbled thoughts I began to pray. "Take this burden, Lord; I cannot bear it! My precious son—I gave him to you, Lord. He belongs to you. Love him. Keep him close to you. Keep him from sin and evil. . . ." I couldn't put my emotions into words. The enemy began pelting me with doubts and guilt. "Where have I failed? Haven't I prayed for him a thousand nights? Didn't I model Christian principles? Didn't I affirm him in his gifts? Why me? Our only son. . . ." A million thoughts raced through my mind, leaving me weak and shaken.

How will Marvin accept this news? How can I protect him? I must be brave. I mustn't show my grief to my husband. I have to make everything better. . . .

I must hurry with dinner as he'll be home soon. I couldn't remember what my plans for lunch were. Numbly I grilled hamburgers, heated leftovers, and put out some fruit when I heard his footsteps in the utility room. Quietly I prayed, "Please protect him from anger and blame. Give him an unusual measure of love!"

"What's in the mail?" he asked as he entered the kitchen, tossing his cap on a chair.

"It's on the table," I mumbled, then promptly left the kitchen, almost in a daze. I wished it were a dream, that it wasn't true. My mind couldn't compute the new information.

As I slowly moved back into the kitchen, the pages from the letter fell to the table. Marvin's face clouded as he said, "Well, I'm not surprised."

I caught my breath sharply. "I'm glad he felt free to tell us, and I'm glad for his expression of love," I ventured timidly.

We sat down and made a pretense of eating, both of us silent. As I picked at my food, my mind backtracked to the day Roger wrote us from Boston informing us of his decision to go to California. Chills raced up and down my spine even now as I recalled the unrest at Berkeley, the hippie movement, strange lifestyles, and demonstrations against the traditional. How I feared for him! It was as though a cloud of doom overshaded our aspirations for him. We could not, however, allow him to know our fears, and would wish him well.

Roger graduated from Goshen College, Goshen, Indiana, with a degree in Social Welfare and accepted a position with the Elkhart County Social Rehabilitation Services. He worked with old age assistance and dearly loved the elderly. He spent hours off-duty assisting his senior friends.

He had so much compassion for the needy, the disadvantaged, the poor, the neglected, the abused, and the retarded.

Some of Roger's friends were pursuing further education in the Boston area, and he made a decision to join them and find employment there. He found a job at Fernald's, a state school for the retarded, and was put in charge of a group of the most severely handicapped adult males. He gave loving care to these "friends," as he called them, for 18 months before deciding to go to California.

The burden of his future lay heavy upon me as I tried to put the pieces of the puzzle together, but my emotions were raw and deep, almost like a death sentence. How big was my faith? Could God keep him from evil?

Again and again I went back to the Scriptures, especially Psalm 31.

> In you, O Lord, I have taken refuge;
> let me never be put to shame;
> deliver me in your righteousness.
> Turn your ear to me,
> come quickly to my rescue. (1-2)

Failing in strength and wounded in spirit, I made it through the day, claiming Jehovah God as my refuge, as a place to hide.

After a long, warm tub bath, I found my way to bed. Marvin was already apparently asleep. How could he be sleeping so peacefully with our world shattered? I wondered.

Sleep eluded me . . . 11:00 . . . 12:00. . . . Again I recalled the words of David and identified with him:

> Be merciful to me, O Lord, for I am in distress;
> my eyes grow weak with sorrow,
> my soul and my body with grief.
> My life is consumed by anguish. (9-10)

The months and years of our life with our dear son Roger, the middle of our three children, paged across my mind. I remembered only the good times . . . the joy he brought us . . . the pride we took in his achievements . . . his love for music. I recalled his first vocal solo when he was three years old at a large family reunion. He was applauded as a future star. Roger was so gifted.

We tried not only to teach but to model values and ideals based on our Christian faith. As a child he loved to hear Bible stories at bedtime, and especially the story of Joseph. When I read the part of being rejected by his brothers and sold to merchants of Egypt, his eyes would fill with tears.

"Shall we read another story?" I'd ask.

"No, read more," he would reply. Why would he want to hear a story that always made him cry? I knew then that somehow he identified with the "least of these." The Danny Orlis series on the radio was also a favorite with him, and the pioneer stories of Laura Ingalls Wilder held a special charm.

I remembered the sweet sorrow as we watched him pack his car and leave for college some 950 miles distant. He had always added spice to our everyday living, and we'd miss his ready smile. After a long hard workday, he'd relax under the large spreading oak with his guitar, singing his heart out. Sometimes the clusters of stars in the black night sky were his only audience. Sometimes it was the piano that gave rise to his emotions. Always it was therapy—and it was beautiful. How quiet our world would be without him!

I remembered the inspiration I had on Mother's Day to pen him a love message in May 1970:

To My Son on Mother's Day:

One night I lay in a hospital bed breathing deeply and yearning for the end, for daybreak to give life to a healthy baby for whom we had prayed and whom we had already dedicated to God. What Thanksgiving when that precious bundle was put into my arms—and it was a boy.

A hundred nights I asked myself in panic, "Is he still breathing?" and would hurry to your bed and touch your soft, warm body. I anxiously worried, "Does he have pyloric stenosis?" when repeatedly you would regurgitate your formula.

On sunny afternoons you stood in your bed and reached for a sunbeam. I would watch you chase a butterfly, stopping in disappointment to watch it soar higher and higher, far out of your reach. Lovingly you would pick a wild flower or dandelion and bring it to me as only a child's heart of love could do, and I secretly wept in thanksgiving for such a loving deed.

I read you bedtime stories. You always wanted me to read the story of Joseph. Sometimes I could detect a tear as you identified with Joseph's rejection by his brothers. I knelt by your bed and listened to you pray.

I have heard your cries when your little bare feet stepped on a sand-burr or piece of glass. Through the childhood illnesses, I stroked your head and held your hand and prayed in concern.

I have looked at school pictures of disheveled children and seen only one face—yours. I sat in auditoriums from grade school to your college years where among a hundred performing children, only you stood out.

I have watched you at play with strange children when you stood aside, shy and frightened.

I have gone at the tug of your hand to inspect tent houses, your tree house or a snow fort. Always it was mother's day.

I have scolded and chastised and paddled. I have laughed, applauded, and advised. I sewed a bag for a camping kit, helped you gather firewood for a campfire, laced your shoes, made milkshakes, baked cookies, packed picnics, and tried to perform the many small joys for you that complicate and enrich a mother's day.

I have screamed at you in impatience over unimportant things and been overwhelmed with forgiveness when you said, "I'm sorry." Then it was Mother's Day.

Dad and I have shared you and delighted in the sharing. There were times of arbitration when we explained you to each other and times you drew apart from me for father's days I could not share. Best of all were days of harmony and fun we enjoyed together—family days. Days we took off and went to Salina, Wichita, or Kanopolis to just be together for fun days.

From the window I have watched you at play and at work developing strength and independence and have felt the tug of having to release you.

I was warmed and touched to see you relax after a hard day's work under a tree in God's great outdoors with your guitar and a song in your heart; or come into the house and hear the piano vibrating violently in response to the emotions of its player.

I have given you over to teachers, leaders, ministers, coaches, professors—and grateful to them for what they gave you of themselves and proud to share my mother's days. Sometimes I have been jealous that always you show them your best face while at home you wore your other faces (realizing of course that this is as it should be).

The world claims you more and more and I go to bed not knowing where you are, but loving you always and entrusting you into our heavenly Father's care. The hardest thing is to just stand aside and watch you take life's stony road.

Now you have grown strong and manly. With courage, confidence, and faith you face the struggles of life. You are *very* special in my heart, but even more special to

God. He's preparing you for a special place. Keep your ear tuned in. Keep love in your heart. Keep your faith strong.

I gave you life, and every fulfilling day you have given me back something wonderful of yourself on a succession of endless mother's days. Thank you and God bless you.

Mom

I began to probe my mind further. How long had Roger struggled with an identity problem? When he was a first-grader his teacher at a parent-teacher conference shared that he had a social maladjustment. She could not define it to us. Could it be that so early in life he had already suffered? I didn't really care to think about it. Then I recalled that he always had a good time with the girls. He liked them and they seemed to enjoy him. He participated in intramural sports in grade school years but he would rather sing or play an instrument than play ball.

I never questioned his interests or activities, as he usually excelled in whatever he did. He took part in all the special music groups and events, earning many medals for superior performance. He was good in art, in debate, and forensics. He enjoyed musicals and plays, usually having lead roles.

Most of the senior boys drove late-model accelerated sports cars and prided themselves in having the biggest and most powerful engines. They sneered and made fun of Roger's older model Falcon, the only heap we could afford to buy for him. I recall one night about midnight, he slammed into the house and rushed upstairs and from his room we heard violent sobbing and crying. Marvin looked out in time to see a car race off into the night. Roger was so broken he could hardly speak as we hurried to his bedroom to find out what had happened.

Finally it came out. Some guys had stopped him after a school function at Inman, where he attended high school, kidnapped his girl, and chased him home. Marvin immediately returned the chase and caught up with them near town. He'd let the fellows know they were identified. I was overwhelmed with grief for my son.

In his first year of college he had what seemed like a serious relationship with a lovely sophomore. He often brought her home and we thought he had made a good choice. She was a Christian and had all the qualities of a good marriage partner. Then one day he told us that the relationship was getting too serious and he needed to break it off. He had too many years of school down the road to support a wife. From then on his friends, including girls, were always just "friends." It is amazing how enduring and lasting those friendships became. Only now did I learn that he was never going to have another serious relationship with any girl. It would only be a dream. For the last 14 years our home had become a place for Roger to visit and remember.

My meditations in the night led me to affirm that purpose and fulfillment are choices. To feel challenged and excited, keeping life full of zest and enthusiasm, is also a personal decision. As we live in the awareness of each day's joys and trials, we can choose the ministering spirit of the heavenly Father, who brings words of encouragement, hope, comfort, and conviction.

"I am claiming that presence tonight, Lord," I prayed. "I'm remembering that David's refuge *never* failed." Accepting that shelter for me personally, I finally drifted off to sleep.

2

A Grave Error

After we regained our balance from the blow, we exchanged letters on a regular basis, always being careful not to address issues that might alienate us from him. The fear of loss always seemed to haunt me. Sometimes Marvin cautioned me in becoming too accepting of Roger's lifestyle, thinking we dare not compromise our understanding of what all that implied. At times I felt I was being squeezed between wanting to please and understand Roger and at the same time wanting to understand Marvin's concern in not endorsing his lifestyle. Couldn't I love unconditionally? My heart was reaching ever so far.

More and more it appeared as though Roger felt free to share what was happening in his life. It felt so good to gain that awareness. His quest for happiness and peace continued.

This is a quote from a letter dated September 2, 1980:

> I auditioned for the Gay Men's Chorus last May and started singing in June. I haven't sung since *The Monterey Peninsula Chorus*, so I was quite out of shape vocally, but my ear and sight-reading skills pulled me through. We are quite professional with over 90% of the chorus having musical training.
>
> It is definitely the most exciting musical organization

I've ever participated in. We sing a variety of music from classical and religious to pop, and we have a large and enthusiastic following here in San Francisco. The San Francisco Conservatory of Music has again invited us to sing in their Schubert Festival this spring. We are now beginning to be recognized outside the gay community by the city and Greater Bay area musical community, as is evidenced by the review we received in this week's *San Francisco Chronicle* following our concert last weekend. Even Mayor Feinstein appeared and spoke at our summer concert, praising and acknowledging us for our excellence and the contribution we are making to San Francisco.

He enclosed pictures taken on rehearsal night and an article by Joan Chatford Taylor from the *Chronicle* dated Tuesday, October 3, 1980, entitled "The Gay Men's Chorus —More Than Music." Taylor reported the following:

"It's finding family," said a second tenor from the Midwest. "When I moved here having left behind a family, I found myself facing the blunt reality of the lack of commitment in a community of singles. A lot of people are just tired of the bar and drug scene.

Each member devotes an established 560 hours a year to the chorus. The schedule and the emphasis in serious musicianship have gradually eliminated the men who joined the chorus thinking it would be a novel way to find new dates."

Roger's letter continued:

Next summer we are going on a national tour. The itinerary is enclosed. I think it will be much fun flying around the country singing. We present seasonal concerts as well as singing at all sorts of events around the country as we are invited. It provides a great opportunity for us as the chorus is really a "family-oriented" group, is very nurturing and supportive in nature, and provides many parties and activities. It's a social connection for a lot of people. . . .

I also am sharing with you some literature from BMC—the Brethren/Mennonite Council for Gay Concerns. You may have already been aware of this organization but if not, I wanted to let you know about it in case you're interested in keeping up with the evolution happening in the Mennonite Church in regard to attitudes around homosexual orientation. I know it is only a matter of time until the church recognizes that we really are all God's children, even those of us who prefer same-sex relationships. I think it is exciting that there is an organization dedicated to increasing the consciousness of the church.

I really want to invite you to avail yourself of any literature, seminars, or discussions which will aid you in becoming educated about homosexuality and examining your attitudes around it. I know we have never really discussed my personal sexuality out of fear on both of our parts. My fear that your interpretation will not allow you to accept that part of me and that you will think less of me somehow. You probably have fears that I will judge you for it, and let it get in the way of experiencing your love for me.

I feel it is really time for us to be without our fears and allow ourselves to more fully understand each other. I want you to know that I *do* understand your point of view and that I don't judge you for it. I also know that any attitude you may have about my sexuality has *no* effect on your love for me. I'm just letting you know that I am willing to budge the door open a bit further and give you the opportunity to do the same.

It seemed good that Roger could find pleasure and fulfillment with a group that recognized his worth and musical talent, so much a part of him. In letters that followed, rehearsals and social activities centering around this group had met a real need. We were glad that he had found a satisfying experience.

We formed plans for his visit home over the Thanksgiving holidays. We were finding more freedom in sharing our beliefs surrounding various issues, yet I felt a bit of caution out of fear in losing his love. I have always believed that we can bridge any differences through dialogue, verbalizing our ideas.

The opportunity came during his visit home. After an evening meal with our entire family, we adjourned to the living room to listen to a tape of the Gay Men's Chorus which Roger had brought along. There was no doubt about it. They were professional! We enjoyed the music. He was so eager for our approval and he so much enjoyed talking about his involvement.

A lengthy discussion about his sexuality followed—that is, between him and me. Marvin and the other kids were absolutely mum. How much I wanted for them to participate in the exchange, but not one word! I was to learn later that their ignorance kept them from taking part. Much of it was new information that they had never processed. It was as though their lips were sealed.

Roger talked about this struggles for identity, his difficulty in meeting the macho image, his inability to cope with heterosexual expectations, and his same-sex preference.

I quizzed him as to when he had come to the realization that he was "different." He related an incident when he was of junior high age and reviewed a number of events during his high school and college career, including a serious relationship with a girl while in college. His behavior seemed traditional and normal to me. Out of the discussion came an awareness of his search for identity and lack of fulfillment in heterosexual relationships. A deep feeling of sadness inundated me and my heart cried out for him. How could we make things better for him?

Yet the family remained quiet. Were they not listening? Why am I doing all the talking? I frantically asked myself. They were too numb to speak and confessed later that they felt absolutely tongue-tied. The information was so baffling. They could not handle it. Evidently they had not thought about it as long as I had, I decided.

Roger gave us posters and information about his upcoming summer chorus tour and solicited our attendance at the Lincoln, Nebraska, concert. I sensed Marvin's reluctance and put him off, saying we would discuss it and let him know later.

One March 3, 1981, we received a letter:

> Just wanted to send you this literature on the chorus. We're putting a lot of publicity out these days as we approach national tour time. We are going to be featured in *People* magazine soon. I'll let you know when so that you can pick up a copy. I really hope you'll be able to come to Lincoln to hear us. We are going to be doing all the best music we've ever performed and it's going to be a *wonderful* concert!

Several phone calls followed as the concert tour date approached. Each time he encouraged us to come. He so much wanted our approval or attendance. The deadline came and we had to give an answer. Marvin felt very strongly that our attendance would indicate our approval of the homosexual lifestyle and he could not do that. I was fearful of jeopardizing our relationship, but saw no other recourse than to say we weren't coming and would give detailed reasons by letter.

I prayed for wisdom and discretion in writing that letter. I so much wanted to please him and I was so fearful that he would not understand our position. I spent several days writing the letter and I believe that what I wrote came from God. I sent it in the hope and prayer that he might understand. But I was *totally wrong*!

We received the following reply May 9, 1981, the day before Mother's Day:

Dear Dad and Mom:

Your letter hurt me so deeply that I am going away from you to heal. I have never been so totally put down in my entire life or had my self-esteem so damaged. At this time I cannot relate to you on any level and I don't even want to discuss it.

Don't include me in the circle letter anymore and don't call. I have absolutely nothing to say to you.

Roger

There are no words in the English language that can convey the anguish, regret, and sorrow I felt! A thousand nights my pillow was drenched with tears before sleep could finally come. Sharing that letter was certainly not worth breaking off our relationship with our much-loved son. Why was I led to write it? Had I not listened to the Lord's counsel? I grew angry with God and cried out for mercy.

Wash away all my iniquity and cleanse me from my sin. Restore to me the joy of your salvation and grant me a willing spirit, to sustain me.

The sacrifices of God are a broken spirit; a broken and

contrite heart, O God, you will not despise. (Psalm 51:2,
12, 17)

Could I ever forgive myself? Could I ever recover our
son's love? Would he ever reach back? What could I do
to regain his respect—let alone his love? If ever I needed
someone to cry with it was now! Could I ever bring
myself to share this burden with anyone? The searching,
the praying, and the anguish went on for days, weeks,
even months.

After six weeks, I started writing to Roger, just news
about family and local happenings. No ideas, just small
talk. How much I longed for a word, a postcard, anything. How sorry I was for the way I'd hurt him! I could
never recall the words I had written. Hadn't he read the
words that told him how much we loved him?

I continued to write regularly. Day by day I turned
over my anxieties to the Lord and trusted him to bring
about a healing in our relationship. Finally one day four
months later, he sent a letter informing us of a change
of address and briefly summarizing his activities of the
past few months. What treasured news. It was *wonderful!* The silence was broken. The Lord was beginning to
answer our prayers.

Brief letters began to come. A phone call brought the
news of his intended trip to Bali, Indonesia. How good it
felt to finally be speaking with each other again. Would I
ever be able to ask for forgiveness for the offense I had
caused? Yet to mention it would only open up the
wound. I had to be certain before another attempt that
might end in failure.

Through these experiences I struggled with grief and
tried to cling to the assurance of God's love. I found
many of my feelings and hopes mirrored in Scripture,
for example, in Lamentations:

Because of the Lord's great love we are not consumed, for his compassions never fail.

They are new every morning; great is your faithfulness
. . . .

Though he brings grief, he will show compassion, so great is his unfailing love.

For he does not willingly bring affliction or grief to the children of men. (Lamentations 3:22-23, 32-33)

3

The Prophecy

One beautiful, quiet sunny summer morning in August 1981, I was on sick leave from my employment as director of nursing services at The Cedars, an intermediate care facility for 69 persons located just two blocks from our home. My body had broken under the stresses of living. It was difficult to hire and maintain quality care-givers for residents with such a variety of needs. I had a deteriorated disc in my back and the doctors prescribed a four-week rest period. The concern for Roger was always before me. How difficult to wait on God's timing! I had faith to believe that God would answer our prayers, but I found myself bringing the burden back and feeling its heaviness.

I turned again to the Psalms: "Commit your way to the Lord; trust in him. . . . Be still before the Lord and *wait* patiently for him . . ." (from 37:4, 7; emphasis mine).

On this particular morning I felt unusually lonely. It would be a long day. Marvin had appointments and would not be home for lunch. How often I had wished for a day of rest with no responsibilities. Now that I had it, I really didn't appreciate it at all.

I was reclining in my chair when the doorbell rang. To my delight my dear friend Betty was at the door.

"It was such a beautiful morning that I decided to do

some biking," she lilted. "I hadn't planned to stop here, but as I went by, I suddenly felt that I was supposed to stop, so here I am!"

I drew her indoors. "And I really needed you today!" I exclaimed.

I was already encouraged because she has such a contagious, bubbling personality. She has, among other things, the gift of making things better. I already knew I was in for a treat.

I told her about my health problem and we soon got on the subject of how the Lord deals with us. Releasing our anxieties and burdens seemed easier talked about than actually practiced. We began thanking and praising the Lord, naming many ways in which we saw him at work in our lives. It was such a joy to rehearse happenings and how we later saw God's hand in it. As we read the Scriptures the words came alive.

Then followed a time of prayer, Betty and I taking turns leading audibly as things came to our minds. Our prayers turned to Roger. We thanked God for what he was doing in him. Being able to praise meant that I was accepting the fact that God was somehow working out his purpose. I wanted to be joyful and trusting for I had dedicated Roger to God.

And so I prayed and thanked God, in accord with Paul's exhortation in 1 Thessalonians 5:16-18: "We know, Lord, that you love us and you love our son even more than we do. We're going to trust you that you're working in his life for what you know is best for him. We praise you for applying your wisdom to his fractured life and for your love toward us."

The more Betty and I prayed, the more we became convinced that God was indeed doing what was for the best. Hadn't God allowed Satan to harass Job and afflict him because he loved God? God allowed the darkness and evil forces of this world to gain an apparent victory—apparent to our senses—yet all the while God's perfect plan for the salvation of the world was being worked out.

Betty started praying in her prayer language and I felt the presence of the Lord so very real, as though he was present in person beside us. Suddenly her voice changed and the following words poured out: "Daughter of Zion, because of your faith, your beloved son, Roger, my rebellious child, will come to me. He will walk in obedience and he will be a witness to me all the days of his life."

Her praying continued in tongues for a short time. I was overwhelmed with love, assurance, and peace. God indeed had spoken! He *would* bring about his will in due time. I believed it!

What a time of rejoicing we had! Betty was not aware of the words of the prophecy, but I well remembered them. They became my source of praise. She then gave me additional words of promise and comfort from Jeremiah 31:16-17:

> This is what the Lord says:
> "Restrain your voice from weeping and your eyes from tears,
> for your work will be rewarded," declares the Lord.
> "They [Roger] will return from the land of the enemy.
> So there is hope for your future," declares the Lord.
> "Your children [Roger] will return to their own land [God's territory]."

By now morning had turned to midafternoon. My visitor had turned into a heavenly messenger. I had felt the presence of God and the assurance of his words. I had experienced the fellowship of his Spirit. She had truly been my encourager.

I was expecting the miracle—and *soon*! I had yet to

learn that my time was not God's time. During the days and months that followed, the message was our hope and we continued to believe it.

4

A Dark Day in August

The months and years dragged by. One warm, lazy August Saturday in 1985, Marvin and I prepared for Sunday as usual. He had been given the responsibility for maintaining the lawn at our church, and Saturdays called for last-minute grooming. He reveled in the relaxation and satisfaction of seeing that it was well-cared-for. For most of his productive years Marvin had been a farmer and also owned and operated earth-moving equipment. He practiced soil conservation and built many terraces, waterways, and dams. Before leaving the farm he had studied and passed exams which qualified him for selling real estate and all types of insurance. He was now associated with a local real estate and insurance firm. Although he enjoyed his sales experience, he liked to operate the church's small tractor and Grasshopper Mower.

I had cleaned the house for guests or unexpected drop-ins over the weekend, which called for some extra preparations in the kitchen.

We had finished our Saturday chores and were relaxing in our den when the telephone rang. The call was from Roger in San Francisco, and we both were on the line. It was always so good to hear Roger's voice. He had been calling more frequently. He said he'd been ill.

We had last seen him when he came home for Janene's wedding the previous November. Janene, our third child, was just two and one-half years younger than Roger. She and her husband, Bob, a food salesman, lived in Salina.

Roger had appeared thin but claimed to be in good physical condition. He was so eager to share his experiences from his month-long vacation to Bali, Indonesia, just six months prior to his visit with us. He brought a larger portfolio of pictures he had taken, and we listened as he told about each picture. He had enjoyed it so very much, he said. He would never be the same because of it. We asked him what it was about the experience that made it so meaningful.

His eyes lit up. "It's the *people*! They're so genuine and loving. They love you because of who you are, not for your accomplishments, wealth, or prestige. They have an honest concern for you and your welfare. They have joy and satisfaction in their families and just enjoy one another."

It puzzled me a little. Is that not the way we are, I wondered? Was he feeling alienated from us in our concept of who he was? I remembered his search for identity. After going to California he was intent on that search. He enrolled in the University of Man and took courses on finding his identity. He also enrolled in the Erhart Training Seminars, to gain affirmation of who he was.

I was deeply disturbed when I learned of his quest, for I had yet to discover the meaning of it all. Verses from Scripture rolled through my mind: "You will know the truth, and the truth will make you free" (John 8:32, RSV). The application seemed so difficult for him. I didn't verbalize my thoughts. I asked only for wisdom to know when to speak. Of one thing I was certain: I didn't know the struggles of what it is to have a homosexual orientation. Later, I was to learn that most of these persons don't plan to be homosexual; instead, it's sometimes a painful discovery they make at one point or another in their lives. Their decision, then, is whether they will resist the perceived homosexual orientation, be celibate, or express that orientation in same-sex relationships. The relational and psychological pain some people experience is incredible. I had yet much to learn.

I recalled that once Roger had experienced the freedom found in accepting Jesus as Savior when he was 12 while attending a junior high camp at Divide, Colorado. What a good time he had! The experience was real and meaningful. The bus in which he traveled, along with thirty-five other young people, arrived home at 4:00 a.m.

He bounced into our bedroom early that morning and announced, "Guess what happened to me at camp!" Not waiting for an answer, he burst out, "I accepted Jesus as my Savior!"

We were delighted and overjoyed with the news.

But in the years and succession of events he had lost sight of the joy of that experience. The complexities of life had taken their toll and blurred his grasp of who he was.

His eyes were sad as he related his reluctance to leave Bali and its lovely people. "I'm planning to go back next fall," he announced.

I could tell that he wished he could make it more clear to us. Obviously we couldn't begin to understand what he felt. And he was unable to express these feelings.

On this visit we expressed concern about his health. We knew that, among other things, he had suffered a serious bout with hepatitis, but he assured us he was well.

I recall his tender good-bye and the warm sadness in his eyes as we took him to the airport. There was something different, some reluctance in leaving us. This moment was very special to me. We took some last-minute pictures at the airport which we treasure highly.

That August Saturday when he called, after some brief greetings on the telephone, Roger said, "I just came back from seeing the doctor, and he shook his head and said, 'There's nothing more that I can do.'"

Together we reviewed his medical history. He had developed a series of infections since January, and had worked part-time until March 1, when he was no longer able to work. From time to time he would call for advice or information, relying on my skill as a nurse. It seemed he had already done everything I suggested. He had sought help from one specialist after another.

My mind roiled with depressing ideas; always I would push my anxieties into my subconscious, for I could not deal with them.

Finally I blurted out, "It seems so strange to me that you have all these infections, one right after another, and you never get over one until another serious problem appears."

Then came his overwhelming response: "Well, Mom, I don't have an immune system!"

My breath came in short gasps. "Do you have . . . AIDS?" I choked out.

I wanted to hold my ears shut so I couldn't hear his answer, but I already knew.

"Yes." The word sounded deep and sad, like a death knell.

A long discussion followed, the contents of which I never really heard. There was no immediate response from Marvin, who was in the den on the other phone. I could only hear his deep breathing.

"Do you want us to come out?" Marvin finally asked.

"No, not now. It isn't the right time," Roger muttered.

I stood numb, my hands cupped to my face. It can't be true, Lord. I must have misunderstood! Why is this happening to us? Haven't we suffered enough? Have we not prayed for our only son night and day to be protected from sin and evil, and to find himself in your will and purpose? Haven't we been faithful?

A thousand thoughts raced helter-skelter through my mind, and none of them made sense.

Marvin suddenly stood in the dining room doorway. "I think we'd better go out right away."

I agreed but couldn't seem to put into words what I was feeling. My mind and emotions had gone crazy. I must be in control, I reasoned.

"I think so too," I said weakly when I could collect my thoughts.

Marvin suggested we call our oldest daughter Sheryl and family, and Janene and Bob, invite them over for Sunday dinner, and let them help us make a reasonable and wise decision.

After sharing the startling, overwhelming news with them, I made plans for Sunday dinner. The wheels of my mind kept turning over and over. I knew very little about AIDS. One thing I knew for certain: it was fatal. At that time news and data about the disease were scarce. I had read a few news clips, a little information in nursing journals, and heard some statistics on TV. Until now I had no personal interest or reason to study it. Suddenly a thought hit me: if we plan a visit, what precautions do we take? Is it contagious?

Sunday morning Marvin and I were in Sunday school and church as usual. It was a difficult morning. I couldn't control my tears, and I thought I would explode. I couldn't conceal that awful secret inside me, and I had to share it. But who would ever understand? Would blame be pointed at us? It didn't seem to matter. I needed someone to help carry the burden. Wasn't that what friends were for?

We were part of a small group that met every Sunday morning before worship in our Mennonite church. Boldly yet tearfully we shared our sad news with our confidants as we told them of our plans to take a hurried, unexpected trip to San Francisco to see our son who was terminally ill. Immediately they surmised it was cancer.

With trembling lips I blurted out the truth. "No, he has AIDS."

A stunned silence followed briefly.

Yet the love response we experienced at that time carried us through the following days, weeks, and months. Had we not been able to share it at that time, I don't know how we could have survived. No value can be placed on the worth of Christian friends.

Around the dinner table that Sunday we made plans for an immediate visit to San Francisco. Leo and Sheryl decided that we needed support and they would take us west in their new Ford Tempo; the cost of four airline tickets was prohibitive. Leo, who was president of a local bank, would consult his board for a week's leave.

We decided to tell Roger of our plans. Marvin dialed the number and we waited for his eager response, telling him the events and plans of the past 24 hours.

"I wish you wouldn't come," Roger's tone was sullen.

"But we just want to see you and share our love with you," Marvin said.

"It's best that you come later. The time isn't right, now," Roger insisted.

"I don't think we can stand *not* to come," Marvin said. "We just have to see you. Leo and Sheryl have made plans to bring us in their Tempo. Okay?"

After a brief silence, "Okay," came Roger's reluctant reply.

With mixed emotions I began to pack for the trip. We planned to arrive in San Francisco about noon on Wednesday. Leo would fly home on Sunday and we would leave by car on the following Wednesday, arriving home on Friday.

5

Unwelcome Guests

Four o'clock Monday morning we packed our suitcases in the car along with an air mattress and extra pillows bound for a journey into the unknown. How much we needed the care and provisions of our heavenly Father! We claimed the promise of the psalmist: "Commit your way to the Lord; trust in him and he will do this" (37:5).

Friends and family had assured us of their prayers and the promise that God would go before us and be our fortress and refuge. With renewed courage and anticipation we left the plains of Kansas behind and headed toward the mountains.

After eighteen long hours we pulled into a Motel 8 for a few hours of rest. At 5:00 a.m. we again pushed on toward our destination. Fourteen more hours through the desert and over mountain ranges found us ready for rest and sleep. We wished we could shrink the miles between us. Our minds and thoughts never ceased quizzing for answers to our many questions. How would we find Roger? How sick was he? Could he walk? In what condition would we find his apartment? How had he been able to function alone? Would he appear very frail? How contagious was AIDS, really? Would his friends accept us? On and on unanswered questions bombarded us. It was difficult to engage in any other topic of conversation. Always it went back to Roger.

After another four hours of driving we approached San Francisco. In the midst of this mad six-lane traffic going full speed, how could we slow down enough to read highway directions? Would we ever find Diamond Street in hills so steep we felt we were falling backward while climbing?

Knowing we were in the general area, Leo stopped to ask for directions. What a thrill to see the street sign, *Diamond.* But would this little car ever make it to the top of the hill? When we quit climbing the road seemed to stop. Not until the front wheels dropped over the edge could we see the road below us. This was a roller-coaster experience to people who live on the plains! We saw beautiful Victorian architecture and the house numbers told us that we were within a block of Roger's house. Suddenly there it was. We immediately saw there was no parallel parking but cars were parked heading into the curbs to keep them from rolling.

We sat for a moment in silence, reflecting. There was almost a hesitancy, as the question seeped into each of our minds: what was waiting for us? Finally we got out of the car and approached the gate to the double-locked entrance. The gate was open and Marvin punched the doorbell three short rings—which was to become our code.

After a long wait which seemed an eternity, the door opened. I was not prepared for the pathetic figure that stood before us. One by one we were greeted with an affectionate hug, and it was hard to hold back the tears. The tall, gaunt, very frail figure that stood before us, a beard about one inch in length with a scaly skin condition all over his body, was our dear son! With a cane in one hand and hanging onto furniture with the other, he led the way to his bedroom and bed.

I sat on the bed and the others found chairs around it. We exchanged cordial greeting and he updated us on his general situation. It was good to see him, but his condition was heartbreaking. In spite of the lush-appearing plants around him and throughout the apartment, there was a cold, distant feeling. A large, ugly mask with long hair, dangling from the ceiling in his dining room, didn't help matters either. Why would he have such a grotesque thing on display? No one dared make a comment.

Roger nervously attempted to fluff his pillow and appear to have a sudden increase of energy. His words became a jumbled mass of conflicting feelings?

"Why did you come? . . . I'm so angry you came. You shouldn't have come. I was so upset about your coming that my therapist had to give me some guidelines and he said I would just have to make some rules. . . . You didn't need to come to try to save me. I have my own beliefs. They may not be like yours but they suit me. . . . I have enough *guilt*. . . ."

By this time I was so broken that I cannot remember the conversation but the word "guilt" came out a number of times. His voice was trembling, his hands shaking, and his eyes glassy and starry-eyed. No one else said a word. There was a long pause.

I was struggling and could no longer fight back my tears. Finally I blurted, "I'm glad you can tell us how you feel and are able to express it. I am just so very sorry that you feel that way. But we came just to love you and share that love with you. I had hoped that all our yesterdays could be forgotten and that we could begin anew today."

His countenance changed and he nodded in agreement. "Where are you going to stay?" he demanded. "There's no room here."

We immediately knew that we would not be using the inflatable mattress. For the next thirty minutes we speculated on where we might stay. He said there were no good motels in the area and we would have to drive back to Highway 101 and closer to the airport to find some. He even made a few calls of inquiry, but without success.

If ever I prayed for guidance it was now. I must be dreaming! This can't be for real, I thought. Why would God allow us to come all this way only to turn around and go home? I went to the bathroom, took authority in the name of Jesus, and prayed that Jesus would be present and real and any darkness of spirit would be overcome.

As I looked around, it was obvious that Roger was no longer the housekeeper. It was totally out of character for his clean, well-ordered, and tastefully decorated home to look like this. The coffee table beside his bed was crammed with medicine bottles, ointments, and tubes of medication, thermometer, and vitamins. Crowded in the middle of it all was a glass dish of snacks: candy, raisins, nuts, and dried fruits. A list of medications stuck out among the bottles. On the bedside stand were fruit, high-caloric drinks, and water.

His telephone, which was his lifeline to the outside world, was cradled on top of the piles of covers along with his Day-Timer. As I glanced at it I wondered how it could be scheduled so full when he was confined to bed. I had forgotten that he was a person given to detail. In it he kept close vigil of all his volunteer helpers as well as appointments.

After a quick survey of the kitchen, I found clean dishes in the dish drainer, a stove that needed some cleaning and a refrigerator with many paper sacks with parts of half-eaten lunches. He had signed up with "Open

Hands," a service founded by Ruth Brinker which supplied meals to 165 AIDS patients. Each evening volunteers delivered a warm meal and lunch for the next day, consisting of sandwiches, fruit, and dessert. A minimal fee of $4 was paid for two meals plus delivery. What a great service to one who is bedfast and living alone!

The sun porch back of the bedroom turned out to be a catchall for the things his helpers didn't know where to stash.

Marvin and Leo decided we needed to leave if we were to find lodging for the night.

"Mom, before you leave I'd like to ask you to do something for me, if you would," Roger said wistfully.

"Of course, if I can," I said. "What is it?"

"I'd like for you to rub my back."

I nodded. "I'd love to."

"There's some vanilla oil on my stand that my masseur uses."

I started unwrapping covers. We learned later that he could never get warm enough. He was wearing sweats, had a woolen blanket on the bed, and two afghans were draped around him. He always carried with him and wrapped himself up in his "security blanket," the brightly colored afghan which I had made for him. The thermostat was turned up much too warm for us. He also had a little electric heater next to his bed and one in the bathroom.

What an opportunity! I was not only going to rub his back but I was anointing with oil. I recalled the promises of James 5:3-16 for healing and forgiveness after anointing and prayers of faith.

Every stroke was a prayer. I could feel his body relax, and I thanked the Lord for what he was going to accomplish through this strange turn of events, a mystery too deep to understand.

When we got up to leave Marvin said, "What time do you want us to come back?"

"I don't know. Call back at six and I'll tell you if I'm too tired to see you."

He may never want us to come back, I thought. My body wanted to groan and I felt nauseated. Sheryl and Roger, though four years apart in age, always related well to each other. Throughout childhood and adolescence they had developed a strong bond between them. They grew up playing in tree houses and snow forts. They played in the creek, made mud pies, and found crawdads. Roger enjoyed learning to cook, build a campfire, or plan a picnic. Duties attributed to housekeeping were often more fun than repairing a motor for the tractor with Dad. I felt she was remembering too.

About six to eight blocks from Diamond we turned on Market Street. Within a few blocks was a big motel sign. It was a large complex with good accommodations, so we decided to stop and sign in.

The day was near perfect, the sun was warm, the breeze cool. Adjacent to our room was a large deck with lawn furniture, tables, and chairs. It was a suitable place to rest and relax.

When Marvin called Roger at six to find out what his wishes were concerning our visit for the evening, he said he was too tired to have us come that night. We could return about nine o'clock in the morning.

I cannot put into words the sorrow that crushed me. I thought I was going to burst.

"If I ever needed a pastor, it is now," I said, choking back the tears.

I put in a call to our pastor Ed at home. He was out of town. But he had given me an address and phone number for the pastor of First Mennonite Fellowship of San Francisco, Ruth Buxman. Upon inquiry he had been told that she was a delightful, committed Christian. I immediately called her. Imagine my joy when she told me that she knew about Roger.

"A member of my church is related to a good friend of Roger's," she said. She volunteered to come to our motel.

We recognized her right away as she approached the stairway to the deck where we were seated. Her genuine warmth and love touched our hearts and gave us comfort. She was so helpful in advising us what to expect and the probable difficulties that Roger had to face in meeting us for the first time since his illness. She affirmed us in our desire just to love him, touch him, and let him know that we cared deeply for him. Before she left, she counseled and prayed with us. To us she was an angel of light. We will never forget her.

After we learned more about the weird environment in which the motel was located, I almost grew panicky. We needed God's promise that he would not let us be tempted beyond our strength and would provide a way for us to make it through (1 Corinthians 10:13).

Marvin and Sheryl were hanging onto the banister of the large deck and had watched the sinister goings-on down the street. There was an open-air cafe several doors from us, and they saw gay behavior, strange to their eyes. A few doors farther we noticed a big sign, Church of Satan. Within this same block was a store with only occult supplies. It was as though we could "feel" the darkness around us! Why, Lord, did you bring us here? I cried. We later learned that this motel was especially active on weekends.

Where could we go for a bite to eat? We weren't hungry, but a cup of coffee would be wonderful. We could not leave by car since there were no parking places. We walked to a large Safeway store a few blocks away and picked up some cereal, milk, and fruit for breakfast. We found a small Greek cafe several blocks from our motel and stopped for a light lunch, ordering a sandwich and a cup of very strong coffee for a dinner price. We had no desire to stay longer than necessary. It was obvious we didn't belong there.

Back at the motel, I decided to call a very close friend of Roger's. Perhaps she could offer some courage and help.

"You shouldn't have come," she snapped. "You've always tried to run his life and tell him what he should and shouldn't do. You've tried to make choices for him!"

My heart was palpitating so loudly I could hear its pounding. If only I could have chosen for him, I thought, life would be much different. How had we chosen for him, I wondered?

I tried to steer the conversation toward her, and expressed my appreciation for her love for Roger and the tremendous help she had given him in so many ways since his illness.

The conversation ended on a friendly note, but with much heaviness in my heart. I didn't expect it to be *this* hard!

Marvin was skeptical, fearing Roger might ask us to leave. I had faith that there was purpose in our coming and I believed in the faithfulness of God.

After showers, we went to bed, but sleep didn't come. The wild, hilarious racket of our entertainers next door and outside on the deck finally settled down and in the early morning our tired bodies gave in to fitful sleep.

6

Love Made Visible

Morning dawned crisp and clear. Rather wearily we got up. After showers we breakfasted on cereal, warm milk, and some fruit, and turned to the Scripture for guidance.

We received comfort as we paged through the Psalms, knowing in our hearts that God is faithful and has promised to help those who trust him and walk in obedience. It was a time for soul-searching. Texts we found speaking to us were Psalms 102:2 and 115:11.

How thankful Marvin and I were for Sheryl and Leo's presence. They were such support for us. It seemed as though my strength was gone, my ability to think and plan blurred. I reminded the Lord that I thought I was tempted beyond endurance . . . yet he had promised he would not test us more than we could bear. We took turns reading, weeping, and praying, each attempting to be strong for the other. There was an awareness of the presence of God and a sense of his abiding Spirit. What blessed peace to experience that! It was with assurance that we left for Roger's house.

Not having a key, we rang the doorbell and waited endless minutes for him to get to the door. He greeted us with a winsome smile and seemed happy to see us. Thank you, Lord, I prayed silently. I *knew* it was going to be a better day, for Roger had planned it.

With paper and pencil, Sheryl jotted down the things to do: grocery shopping, cleaning, laundry, things to be repaired or replaced, etc. Roger had several business errands for Marvin and Leo. He knew that Sheryl was proficient in cleaning and the bathroom desperately needed her touch. My job was basically in the kitchen.

Fried chicken, butterscotch pudding, and cinnamon rolls were on the menu. It was obvious that a trip to the grocery store was one of the first errands. Our efforts in finding a place to park would make a story in itself, but we finally achieved our mission.

Trying to find equipment, pots, and pans to prepare a meal in a kitchen with three feet of counter top seemed next to impossible. I learned that you could use a pint jar for a rolling pin and a pan lid for rolls. I also learned more uses for aluminum foil than I ever imagined, and that one could regulate an oven by turning it off when too hot and on when too cool. I believe the Lord had a hand in making the food turn out palatable.

The aroma of rolls baking was a childhood reminder and brought pleasure to us both. It was amazing to see how things worked together for good. At the end of the day, the rooms sparkled and the scent of furniture polish and wax permeated the apartment. We also gave special care to his plants, prepared three genuine meals, purchased an answering machine, gave several back-rubs, caught up on family news from home, and enjoyed Roger's warm, appreciative spirit.

With the exception of a two-hour rest time, we had spent the entire day following Roger's agenda. We worked quietly, did our best, gave assistance when needed, and responded to questions we could answer.

At our motel room that night, we found the bathroom and shower with about four to six inches of backed-up water and sewage! Not knowing what to do, we called the management. Much later a plumber of sorts came to inspect the complaint. After two hours of cluttering our room with hoses, tools, and buckets we were told to use the small bathroom. It had a shower stall, small lavatory, and stool. Our efforts to clean up were meager at best. Miraculously none of us picked up any "bugs." We thanked the Lord for his protection.

Friday and Saturday we again followed Roger's agenda. Sheryl and I spent a half day washing clothes and bedding. It was obvious that our presence at the laundromat was noticed as out of the ordinary, for we didn't look like typical Californians. We gave the entire apartment a good cleaning. The navy Persian rug in Roger's bedroom was not practical for a patient with a scaling skin condition covering his body. The scales crusted to the bedclothes and to the floor when Roger was assisted to the bathroom.

I spent considerable time scheduling and monitoring his medications. I was appalled at the number of medications he was taking and trying to manage by himself. He would forget or double the dosage, so I set them up on regular schedules and carefully monitored his "give as needed" pain medication. I made out medicine cards to help him in the days to come.

Living alone had become increasingly difficult for Roger. We are indebted to three close friends who assisted with his care since his confinement. Annie, an airline stewardess who lived in the apartment above him, got his breakfast, washed dishes, cleaned, and assisted with his bath. She grocery-shopped and ran many errands for him. Without her help, I don't know how he would have survived. She refilled his drinks and made sure that things were within reach before leaving for work. Rosemary, a friend from college days, was also a trusted confidante. She watered his plants and visited regularly. Ted, also a special friend, took over managing his business, caring for his insurance needs when Roger was no longer able to do so. Without the assistance of these special people he would not have been able to keep going.

While they were willing, it also became very demanding. Unlike most people with AIDS, Roger did not have a live-in friend. We were to find out later that he suffered many feelings of alienation and rejection from the gay community because he felt unsuitable for anyone. How desperately he wanted to be accepted!

Upon arriving at our motel the third night we found the same plumbing problem. The smell drove us back before we even entered. Again we notified the management. After several hours we were advised that it was usable. By now our bodies were tired enough to fall into bed and sleep.

Leo's plane was scheduled to leave at 11:00 a.m. A trip to the airport through unfamiliar territory in hectic traffic confronted us. It was hard to see him leave; he was such a support for us in the upheaval of our emotions. We took turns reading Scriptures, crying, and praying. We could only turn to God for strength and endurance.

> You are my hiding place; you will protect me from trouble and surround me with songs of deliverance. I will instruct you and teach you in the way you should go; I will counsel you and watch over you. (Psalm 32:7-8)

> Fear not, for I have redeemed you; I have summoned you by name; you are mine. When you pass through the waters, I will be with you; and when you pass through the rivers, they will not sweep over you. When you walk through the fire, you will not be burned. . . . For I am the Lord, your God, the Holy One of Israel, your Savior. (Isaiah 43:1-3)

What a comfort and encouragement we received from each other and the Word!

Not knowing if this would be his last good-bye, Leo was concerned about leaving a message of hope with Roger that would not offend him. How and what could he say to him that would be helpful? Marvin wondered if Roger might suggest that we all leave when Leo left. Would we be prepared for that? But I felt more positive and sensed a growing trust in our terminally ill son toward us.

We arrived at his apartment in the morning. Since we now had a key, we identified our arrival with our established code of three short bells. Roger appeared eager to see us but complained of a severe headache. He had forgotten to take his 4:00 a.m. pain medication, and his bedding was drenched in perspiration. He was extremely miserable. I gave him medication at once, fluffed his pillows, and straightened the bedding until bath time could give him fresh, dry linens. Then I fixed breakfast.

Marvin and Leo briefed him on the daily events of our accommodations. Roger felt uncomfortable with our stay at this motel.

You should *never* have gone there," he said, then in the next breath he added, "I just wasn't able to help you and there are no good motels in this area."

He chided us for shopping in the grocery store we had patronized. Besides not being clean, all the bag ladies, pimps, and other riffraff traded there, he told us. He told us where to shop for groceries and which laundromat to use after this.

It was time to leave for the airport, and Leo edged to the bed to give his last words. The rest of us slipped out to other rooms to leave the two alone.

Please God, be in every word; and let it be helpful, I prayed.

"You *will* meet your Maker," I heard Leo say, and I stepped farther into the living room. The conversation was short and I heard Roger's words:

"Thank you so much for coming and being with the folks."

We locked the door and gate and walked to the car in silence. Could we ever engage in meaningful conversation with him again? If only I could know what he is really thinking, I mused. He has so much time for that. He had now been bedfast for nearly six months and had been treated for many infections and bacterial diseases. By now he was wracked with pain and getting noticeably weaker. How could we best convey our genuine love for him?

7

The Greatest of These Is Love

We had learned a routine and each day brought us a bit closer to the purpose of our coming. Marvin had discovered the location of a few vital places: the pharmacy, grocery store, and bank. He had learned to drive with the traffic. But he experienced difficulty with the night errands that took him on Castro Street to the large Walgreen Pharmacy that dispensed many drugs which might be considered unusual for general practice. Castro Street is the center of the gay community.

Now it was our final evening, and we wanted it to be special. I prepared some of Roger's favorite foods. It took me twice as long to fix a meal with all the inconveniences in unfamiliar turf. Although his appetite was poor, Roger praised the food. Of course, none of us were hungry. We choked down the meal and pretended to enjoy it.

We had taken turns at Roger's bedside, sharing words of love and affirmation. We felt that special bonding that happens when soul communion between loved ones takes place. After we had finished supper and dishes, we gathered around the bed for our final visit. Then began a summation of all that Roger had observed during our stay. He lay there, his face hollow and thin, his eyes sunken.

"I want to thank you for all that you did—most of all for your love," he said, his voice husky. "It was as though there were two angels here in the house." He beamed at Sheryl and me, and his eyes shifted from one to the other.

"In your thorough busyness you were so quiet! I saw Sheryl's love in the care and detailed way she cleaned and polished the house and cared for my plants. They look so fresh with clean leaves! I saw Mom's love in the kitchen cooking my favorite foods—the good smells, bread baking, and reminders of home. She showed her care by fixing my medications so that I could be more accurate and seeing that I took what I was supposed to. And her wonderful back rubs!

"I also appreciated Dad's love in his wish to get my business affairs in order, fixing the kitchen sink and drain, selecting a telephone answering service that I wanted, getting groceries, and running errands. Thank you all." His eyes filled with tears and he paused to brush a shaking hand across them. Our emotions didn't allow any of us to speak, yet I was flooded with thankfulness as he went on.

"I know that I'm going to die, and I want you to know I'm ready to die. It may seem that my beliefs are a bit different from yours but they suit me." For the next two and one-half hours he told us his wishes. He expressed his desire to be cremated if it did not offend us, assuming that the practice was not within our Mennonite traditions. He asked us about our plans for our own burial and requested that his remains be buried beside us. What a comforting thought that was! I could hardly believe all I was hearing. He informed us of his business liabilities and assets and his wish for disposition.

He walked back through the beginning of his illness, the fears, struggles, and disappointments he had. He spoke tenderly of the love, care, and support of his friends. What provisions they had made for his comfort! He spoke so fondly of the people and his love for the country, and his eyes lit up as he reminisced about his trip. Annie was going to return to Bali in the fall and he planned to send some assistance with her; they were planning for a joint business venture in merchandising. But most of all, he shared personal messages to those whom he had come to call friends.

He spoke of the regret and sadness that his illness had brought us. He was concerned how it had affected Janene, his younger sister. He wanted us to convey his special love for her.

He grew noticeably fatigued as he continued to talk. Marvin and I hardly spoke. We were eager to carry out his wishes and made it clear to him that whatever he wished we would do our best to carry out. We thanked him for his kindness and for accepting our love and for sharing of himself in the way that he did. Finally we knew it was time to leave.

He reached out a thin, emaciated hand. "Mom, can you give me one last back rub?" he asked.

With tears cutting shiny paths down my cheeks, I nodded. It was so wonderful to give him some comfort and be able to please him this way.

"What do you want us to tell the relatives and friends back home?" Marvin asked when we got ready to leave.

"Tell them to pray for me, and send letters and cards," he said in a tired voice.

It had been a heavy evening, but one we will never forget. It now seemed worth all the discomfort and problems we had encountered. God's love through our touch had spoken. A bridge had been built. We would later learn the impact of this most difficult experience.

We saw to it that his medicines were given and drinks

and nourishment supplied on his bedside table. He wanted the security of his telephone on his bed with the cradle properly placed so that he had an open line if needed. Afghans were in place and lower lights left on. He looked around to check if everything was in order. All that was left was our good-byes. Inwardly I cringed at the thought.

"Thank you for everything," he said as his sad eyes filled with tears.

"Please call us if you need us," I choked out. "If we don't see you again here, we'll meet you in heaven." I gave him a big hug, then turned away to hide my tears.

Sheryl and Dad gave him their teary farewells. We locked the door and gate and walked away into the chilly night.

8

Reflections

Will the pieces of the puzzle ever come together to give a complete picture? Why does God permit the birth of a person who has an identity struggle or who becomes aware of a homosexual orientation? Does it seem fair? Why was Roger among those to feel insecure, misunderstood, shunned, rejected? He did nothing to deserve it. It was not a choice, as I see it.

Roger excelled in so many gifts. He was a very sensitive, tender, compassionate person. He has brought sunshine to so many. His smile was contagious. He treasured his friendships so that they became enduring ones. He appeared to have a happy childhood and enjoyed many friends. Yet the painful discovery made at one point or another regarding his sexual orientation had made a difference and few of us knew of his struggle.

Guilt welled up within me in the days that followed. I began to think of the many things I should have understood, and I sorrowed for my ignorance in the ways I had imposed my beliefs on him. Given another chance, I think I would attempt a more meaningful relationship from a different perspective. At the time I was at a loss to know in what way I needed to change. Didn't I daily seek the Lord and ask for his counsel and direction? Always I was assured of his presence and his faithfulness in bringing to pass his will in his own time and in his own way. How much more patience can I have in waiting for that time? I keep learning and growing in my understanding. Nurturing the inner life became the source of my rest and peace.

Roger's desire to give and receive love was not fulfilling or satisfying to him. He would go to a place where he could immerse himself in a community that loved and accepted him as he was. He did not need to hide his identity there. He would find companionship among others struggling like him. What he needed now was for us to walk with him, not judge him. He was so right. He was miserably involved in fighting a deadly disease—not persons. He needed all the hope and care we could possibly give him for his last days on earth.

What a lonely vigil, while losing everything—all that one ever had or treasured: possessions, friends, family, dreams, hopes and aspiration, and life itself. No one can fully share this journey with another. It is fearful.

Roger's sorrow at not being able to return to Bali lay heavily on him. What really happened to him there that made a difference? I would later learn from his journals. After making stops in Japan and China, his party landed in Sumatra, Indonesia.

While there Roger wrote as follows:

Wednesday, October 6: I woke up at 5:00 a.m., which seems to be becoming a pattern. I felt *so* rested and alive. Went for a walk to look for a few things I needed. Met Steve and Annie for breakfast. We packed, and Jude gave us a ride to catch the ferry for Samosir Island.

The ferry was like a large kayak with a canopy. It was about 45-minute trip from Prapat to the island. We were dropped at Caroline's, which we were told was the best place to stay at Tuk 2. Turned out to be the *perfect* spot for us to spend four days recovering from nonstop travel. It was rest and relaxation time. It's such a relief to not have to think of getting up in the morning and hopping on a bus.

I really need this time to relax, enjoy and assimilate my experiences thus far. Caroline's is a grouping of little batak-style cottages perched on the side of the mountain overlooking the lake. It's just so charming. We decided to splurge and get separate cottages. For $1.50 per night, it wasn't a difficult decision.

My little cottage is quite precious, rustic and gray with a sunny balcony overlooking the lake. A spectacular view! It is extremely peaceful and quiet, except for birds, crickets, etc. It's hard to believe I am here in such a extraordinary spot, feeling centered as I do. It must be heaven!

Got all situated in my room. Picked some fresh flowers, rearranged the furniture, and generally turned it into "home." It's perfect to have my very own space. Was so *contented* to be here with no schedule, nothing I had to do.

Spent most of the afternoon hanging out, writing post cards, reading, etc. Four young men who worked here wanted to be friends. It was so great being with them and noticing the effect their lifestyle here on the island has on their outlook on life. They really live their lives in the "now." So warm, genuine.

Made a lot of headway in adjusting to life here today. Am so relaxed and content. It's hard to recall or relate to the pressures I felt the last few months of the summer. Seems like years ago:

Saturday, October 9: Each day I let go of a little more tension and get a little deeper into the total relaxation.

Each night I sleep a little deeper and wake up feeling more refreshed. Have been doing a lot of deep breathing and "letting go." I had no idea how much tension and anxiety I was carrying around till I landed on this island and began to notice it disappearing.

It's so incredible to wake up 5:00 a.m. and jump out of bed totally alive. Rested! Have been running the past three mornings—a great way to start the day. Road seems best for running toward Tomak. The scene in that the direction is overwhelming. Upon making the turn the first time and catching the view toward mushroom man's house, I thought I was going to pass out.

Water buffalo grazing the slopes keep them manicured like a golf course. Down near the lake, the bright green rice paddies and batak houses complete the scene. It was a long beautiful walk and my head went through incredible space that I can't even write about. Spiritual.

Found several spots for solitude and gazing at the gorgeous surroundings. . . .

Roger related many experiences the following week, adjusting to the customs of another culture, some adventuresome, some frightening, but he always seemed to enjoy the beauty and calm serenity of this island.

On leaving the island: It is so hard to think of leaving here although I am ready to move along to Bukki. This has without a doubt been the most incredible week of my life. It's about letting all of Roger go and just being. It's so refreshing and I just haven't had the opportunity to let go this completely for this amount of time.

It's like having the effect of being in training 24 hours a day for eight days. It's good to be having really warm, positive, and loving thoughts about myself. It's like Annie said about feeling like you are just "inside," no outside exists.

I haven't been able to define all I've been letting go of, but it doesn't matter because it is gone and it is "back there."

It's hard to imagine what the shock of going home will be like. I have given no thought to what I will do with myself back there. I do know that I feel more at peace.

Thursday, October 14: I wish I could explain what all has happened to me here. It has only been the past four or five days that I have been completely relaxed. It took a fair amount of time to get rid of all the San Francisco garbage. It's a new experience to feel my insides smiling all the time. Thank you, Tuk Tuk. It's sad saying good-bye to the gang. Three young men are singing and playing guitar on the small ferry as it pulls in to Caroline's to pick us up. We pull away, the gang waving good-bye for the last time.

Roger told of the 20-hour bus ride to Bukki in an already-packed old bus on a rough, winding road, being tossed about, inhaling intense exhaust fumes, and asking for a "barf bag." They tried to entertain themselves looking at the humorous side of this journey. After delays they finally board the plane at Jakarta.

At one point on the Padang-Jakarta flight I went to the bathroom at the front of the plane. The cockpit door is open. Both pilots are slouched back in their seats, reading, with American disco music blaring away. And who is flying this plane? It is all just too ridiculous.

They finally arrived in Bali.

I got my cottage and it is just *too* perfect. I can't even believe what character it has; thatched roof, bamboo walls, little kitchen area with a bathroom that is open to the backyard. I'm in heaven! I immediately shower, relax for a bit, then take out walking.

He meets many friendly people.

I am moved. I walk on toward the beach. I have to get there tonight. I have no idea where I'm going and hope I don't get lost. I finally reach the beach, run in the water, laugh, kick. It's too wonderful! I lie for a long time on the sand, staring at the stars, listening to the waves. So calming and peaceful. I finally head back to Golden Village, find my way after several wrong turns, and go to bed.

Monday, October 18: I feel ridiculous in thinking already that I won't be able to leave here, considering I haven't even been here for 12 hours yet. I have never felt so immediately in love with any place in my life. The beach is nearly deserted and goes on for miles.

First impression is a paradise surpassing by far my wildest expectations, combined with beautiful and easy inner vibes, making it an experience I can't even begin to write about any more at this point.

Tuesday, October 19: It's so refreshing to find that the gays here are just people, not faggots first as in San Francisco. It's so insignificant, just a preference. No dishing, no macho acts, no competing, no big drug or alcohol trips—just boys who like boys; and more do seem to be boy-types.

Thursday, October 21: I feel so warm, and so in love with everything and everyone and myself that I feel like crying. I believe since coming to Bali it is the first time I have had the experience of crying out of joy. Usually in my life, the times I have cried have been painful times. It's a unique experience to feel tears of joy springing from my soul, gushing out of my physical being. I can't even remember being so happy and at peace with the universe. I cry as I write about it. Moving. Powerful!

I can't believe how my experience of myself back there in the old reality deteriorated. I can't believe how I bought into the phoniness of the gay community. I allowed myself to feel the alienation and to feel myself, but I had no idea how much rubbish had accumulated until it started vanishing and I started feeling all this "space" inside. It's refreshing to know that I will never be the same although it is scary to think of what it will be like to step into my old life, wondering how the new me will cope with my old situation. I don't know how I can live in that environment again. It seems like there is no place else for me to be except here.

I guess the strength I have gained here will empower me to adapt to something new. I love me. I am beautiful and strong and now that I have really had that experience, I know that I can never forget it. I am beginning to realize that I have *never* loved myself. I can't believe how so many years have gone by and how I could have possibly survived all this time without the experience of really loving myself.

So much pain. So little belief in myself. I think the absence of love in my life has been a result of my inability to love myself. I know I have had that thought before but it never meant anything to me because until I *really* had the experience of loving myself, I just couldn't relate to the concept. It didn't mean anything to me.

Every morning and evening the people all make little trays out of banana leaves, fill them with incense, flowers, and food, and put them in front of their doors for the "gods." They are offerings. It is so fascinating. I asked Annie if they haven't figured out that the animals end up eating them, not the gods. She pointed out that they believe that the gods can appear in any form, including animals. They believe that people can turn into animals. Their beliefs in magic, spirits, and the gods are a very real part of their existence. No matter what is actually so on the matter, it is obvious that these people have learned how to live a meaningful existence.

I realize now that the reason I could not sleep for so long last night is that I was building up toward this breakthrough today, whatever it is about. It *has* been a really intense experience for me. It's as though I am at this place and I don't know what to do with myself. I don't know for sure how to be, now that I have learned about loving myself. I also don't know how to write about it, but I do know that as I attempt to describe to myself what is happening, floods of emotion are coming up and it feels really healing to be letting it all out.

I keep moving into more new spaces that are completely new to me. I can't figure out how I have survived so long making life so difficult. I keep thinking this must be it. I must be completely unwound. But more trash from the past just keeps seeping out of my being. I keep experiencing more space inside.

I'm so happy to get acquainted with some locals and get to know more about these people. Madé is so fine. It just amazes me how good he is to us and how easy it is to be around him. He just loves us for nothing and expects nothing in return. You don't have to do *anything* to prove who you are.

It's so exciting, to notice too that somehow people get who I am right away. At home, somehow I always seem to have the feeling that it is such a long and complicated process to get anyone to see who I really am. It's an effort somehow to show them my "insides." Here, somehow, it just happens automatically, almost instantly. No games. No expectations. Just people being completely real with each other.

So often, I have felt that uneasy feeling in being with people for the first time and trying to break through those early social necessities at home. Somehow, it all seems to happen naturally and instantly here. Such connection. Such a relief to feel complete absence of judgment and evaluation. Again, it's a whole new experience for me and sometimes I find myself wondering how we ever got so far away from our ability just to be real with people—without having to prove who we are, or to find some clue that we really can trust them enough for us to be who we are.

Annie is such an inspiration to me. What a beautiful lady she is. It's a treat for me to be with her here, and notice how far she has come in her ability to be instantly genuine. People *love* her everywhere we go. I now understand her so much more—how she has come to be who she is after coming here for seven years. It is profound to watch her be able to transcend all language and cultural barriers and get through to that space of communication that is *real*, that requires no language.

I believe that in the past few days, the stranger and somewhat quiet space I've been in, is due to the fact that I am so overwhelmed by the beauty of life here. I am almost worried about how I can ever cope with San Francisco again! How can I ever walk through the Castro and see all that phoniness and cruelty that exists there? All that cold competition. After having been here and feeling all the warm feelings and affection from friends here, it is so hard to imagine having to go back and work so *hard* to make a real connection with people. Why not be in a place where it just comes natural? Why should I ever have to settle for anything less than this?

Now I have realized that I am beautiful and have for the first time started to see what it is like to really love myself. I realize that I *deserve* being in an environment that reflects such quality.

I am so intrigued with the way they just take you into their lives and open up their souls to you. I think it's a natural ability that we have lost somehow. It is inspiring and so rewarding for me to be able to do the same with them. It is almost magical. It will be interesting to see how I carry this ability when I get back to the "old reality."

I have never felt so totally relaxed, so good about my body and appearance. It's such a switch. Having felt so physically inadequate all my life, I at first felt weird getting all the positive strokes about my body from people here. It's an ego trip to understand that these people think I'm beautiful on the outside as well as the inside.

Amazing, too, that I have spent so little time giving attention to my physical appearance the past month. It's so irrelevant. People here look right through your physicalness; it is unimportant to waste time trying to present yourself in any particular way. So unlike San Francisco, where it seems important to worry about how you look. All that competition.

Madé offered to drive me around Bali on a motorbike. I feel no pressure to see any more of the island this time. It would be nice, but I value just doing the normal daily things. The most important thing to me at this point is simply spending as much time with the locals and absorbing their incredible energy.

There is beautiful scenery everywhere in the world. The interaction that happens with people here, does not happen everywhere. It seems to make sense to take advantage of the more rare opportunities.

Monday, October 25: Had such a great session with Annie yesterday, discussing how it is to live here, how easy it is to feel good all of the time. I'm happy to have been able to contribute to her life by being me and by sharing my insights of the people with her. Talking about it increases our own awareness.

We were talking about sex and how the Balinese don't seem to get into it that much. I have figured out how they don't need to. They are such romantics. They get into the fantasy of "love and romance" so much more than the actual sexual act.

I believe that we have gone to such extremes to experience erotica in order to transcend our reality, to lose ourselves for a short time in that state of bliss. The Balinese are constantly in that state of bliss and it isn't so important for them to get into sex so intensely. They are more into soul stimulation than genital stimulation. To me, it seems so much more natural, more gratifying. Not that sexual bliss doesn't happen for them, but they aren't seeking out the ultimate experience.

It's such peace for me to be here and for the first time feel like I fit in. It is humorous when I think of myself here in a culture so foreign to my own, and get to feeling like I fit in better than at home. I believe I was starting to feel that maybe there was no place on this planet where I belonged. Now I know there is a place where I can just be me and be appreciated for exactly who I am. It's such a relief to have a "spot." It starts to make life worth living.

I realize now how I had descended in my state of happiness and contentment. I suppose as a child I experienced this same state of innocence and happiness, but it has been many years since I have allowed myself to get freely into it. I had forgotten how easy it is to be alive. I am amazed when I remember that a few months ago I could come up with few reasons to go on living. And these reasons were only to spare my family and closest friends the grief of my absence. Now it is all so different as I realize that I want to live for *me*. Not for anyone else, but for the pure enjoyment that I can achieve for myself! I am beautiful inside and out, and I am strong. I am powerful. I know what it is to love and be loved. It makes it all worthwhile.

As I walked to breakfast this morning I just had to smile the whole way. I was meeting Madé, Wyan, Ratus, all of them so glad to see me! Why? How can they seem so exuberant all the time? I feel so at home and so thankful to have had the opportunity to make *real* friends here with real people!

Sunday, October 31: I believe that sometimes the tears of joy have twinges of sadness when I realize how much quality has been lacking in my life. How I failed to see the significance of believing in myself and in other people, the potential for leading a rich and full life. I believe also that part of the sadness comes out of fear—fear that now that I know the endless possibilities of experiencing love, that somehow when I go home I won't be able to incorporate it into my life the way I did in Bali. I don't know how I can ever live without that experience of love in the world of clones. I guess that is my biggest fear of all right now. Now that I know what it can be like to be real with people, all of that competition and sexual emphasis just seems too depressing to ever have to look at—let alone to try to fit into. I fear that perhaps I'm going to feel even more of a misfit than before.

One by one tearful good-byes were said to friends that now seem like forever friends. We made our final stop to say good-bye to Youmand and Madé, the massage ladies. It was a sad and emotional parting; Madé is afraid she will die before we make it back to Bali. And she may. She doesn't look well at all this last day. Youmand is just sweet as ever and goes on and on about how she will miss us.

Annie and I both begin crying again, and we leave soon because it is just too emotional for everyone there. We sniffle all the way to the airport, interspersed with many outbursts of giggling. I regain a certain amount of composure for our one and one-half hour wait at the airport. My mind is just blank, and yet all this emotion is pouring out. I feel so confused about what is happening with me. So sad to be leaving, so elated about what Bali has given me—just a mishmash of emotions.

As we finally take off, I lose it completely. Never before have I been so profoundly affected by a departure. Even at major change times in my life, when I have moved away, leaving many close friends and old ties behind, did not feel so sad and so much mixed emotion. I guess it was that intense because in the last month I have given myself so many opportunities to let go of my emotions completely, to know my feelings precisely, with no holding back whatsoever. It has been so rejuvenating for me to live my life at this level.

I cried nearly the whole way to Jakarta. It was so difficult for me to listen to all the Western tourists on the plane recounting their experiences of Bali and trying to impress others.

It was real shock to get to Singapore and find more of the same. I was in a daze—no one there to look after us, no one being real, no one even connecting with us. In an instant it brought back the icy cold remembrance of life back home. Everyone bustling about in their hotsy-totsy clothes doing their things. I remember the initial shock of landing in Sumatra and how alien I felt. Somehow this is even more intense, because now the shock is a result of seeing evidence of my *own* culture, which now seems as foreign to me as Sumatra did the first day. Where do I fit in *now*?

Oh, dear, dear Roger! Was this the world you felt to be real? Satisfying? Again my heart ached with a physical pain as I was brought face to face with the way he had searched for his personal identity. What had gone wrong with our real world?

9

AIDS Confirmed

AIDS is caused by a virus that attacks the immune system. This leaves the body unable to fight off certain infections and cancers that healthy immune systems destroy with ease. These infections are caused by organisms that most of us already have in our bodies and are commonly found in the environment. When a person develops one of the opportunistic infections or cancers which do not occur in the presence of healthy immune systems, the underlying AIDS can be diagnosed. Other symptoms which may point to AIDS are dementia, loss of appetite, severe emaciation, and dysentery.

For some time Roger experienced symptoms referred to as ARC (AIDS-related complex). Some of these were swollen lymph glands, drenching night sweats, excessive unexplained weight loss, severe chronic diarrhea, severe fatigue, fever, yeast and viral infections in the mouth. He suffered with herpes, candidiasis, hepatitis, cytomegalovirus, and other ailments.

The second stage is the development of an opportunistic infection or of Kaposi's sarcoma (cancer); the latter is characterized by bluish to reddish purple discolorations found on the skin. Lesions can also be found internally, such as on mucous membranes of the mouth, lung, lymph nodes, stomach, and intestines.

The most common opportunistic infection seen is pneumocystis carinii pneumonia. The diagnosis is usually made by bronchoscopy, a procedure in which a tube is place through the mouth into the lungs. More and more we were becoming educated to the nature and treatment of this fatal disease called AIDS.

Telephone calls became more frequent. Gradually he was growing more debilitated, but was determined to fight the disease and was intent on carrying out the best health practices.

One of Roger's many calls came late at night. His sobbing voice was filled with terror. As he cried, "The police are coming to arrest me and take me to jail. I can't believe it's happening to me!"

Dad's first thought was that he had done something irrational that merited the fear, and asked, "What makes you think they will?"

"I have a letter that says, 'If we find your trash in our dumpster again we will call the police. Signed _____ of the _____ Church.'"

In his confusion he was crushed. Dad assured him that he could call when they came and he was sure he could take care of the matter.

Later we learned that the occupants who had just moved into the apartment upstairs, had so much trash they put it along with Roger's into the church's dumpster, which they thought was public. The church custodian had found some letters addressed to Roger.

The cruelty of the world never seemed to end.

Early one Sunday morning in October, 1985, we received a phone call from Goshen, Indiana, informing us that my Aunt Leona had died. We had a special love for her and knew that we needed to make plans for attending her funeral. After numerous calls to family, friends, and Roger, we packed our bags with intentions to leave immediately following the worship service. Was it wise to travel 950 miles east when we might expect a call from California to come west? I will long remember the meaningful worship service that Sunday in which Barbara, a beautiful soprano, sang. "We Shall Behold Him." The anticipation of heaven and being in the presence of Jesus was taking on some powerful significance. Tears flowed freely. Few could know the heavy emotions that gripped us that gorgeous fall morning.

Choosing to drive to Indiana seemed appropriate so we could come and go as we pleased. A possibility for change of plans always surrounded our daily schedules.

It was good to be reunited with family and friends. Though the occasion was sad, the special love and bond that one feels was precious. Our dependency and need for one another had become quite important.

The day following the memorial service for Aunt Leona, the call from California came. Roger was in the hospital. In a soft-spoken voice he said, "I've been very sick. I had to go to the hospital yesterday. The reports came back positive. I have pneumocystis—but I'm going to make it. You believe in miracles, don't you?"

"Yes, I believe in miracles," I said.

Before I could say more, he burst out, "I'm going to be healed. Pray for a miracle. Tell the family there to pray for me. Call everyone and ask them to pray at six o'clock tomorrow evening. I will have some friends here and at that time we'll all pray for a healing miracle. Would you do that?" There was eagerness and urgency in his request.

My heart seemed so heavy in my chest. I could hear it pounding, but I didn't feel panic. I had been under the impression that supernatural healing and deliverance always brings more glory to God and more eternal profit to the individual than continued suffering. But was that what we needed to have faith for *now*? Are there not recorded stories of great saints who made valuable contributions to the kingdom on earth through great suffering, when God chose to withhold a miracle? Hasn't Roger already suffered enough? I thought. Has he not been patient?

Perhaps now God would bring the prophecy to fulfillment. What exciting thoughts raced through my mind! I could think of a hundred ways in which God could be glorified, should he choose to bring healing *now*! Would our doubts hinder healing? James 1:6-7 came to mind:

> When he asks, he must believe and not doubt, because he who doubts is like a wave of the sea, blown and tossed by the wind. That man should not think he will receive anything from the Lord.

My mind was really testing me. Had we lacked faith all these months—even years, as we prayed for healing and wholeness for Roger's body, mind, and spirit? I wanted Job's kind of faith, that did not depend upon tangible fulfillment. "Though he slay me, yet will I trust in him" (Job 13:15, KJV).

When one has weathered testing and trial, he can identify with the author of the following lines:

> I will not doubt, though all my ships at sea
> Come drifting home with broken masts and sails;
> I will believe the hand which never fails,
> From seeming evil worketh good for me.
> And though I weep because those sails are tattered,
> Still will I cry, while my best hopes lie shattered;
>   "I trust in thee."
> I will not doubt, though sorrows fall like rain,

And troubles swarm like bees about a hive,
I will believe the heights for which I strive
Are only reached by anguish and by pain;
And though I groan and writhe beneath my crosses,
I yet shall see through my severest losses
   The greater gain.

(Author unknown)

Our telephone conversation ended on a positive note. We would be in touch. We'd make daily calls and believe God for healing—and an awareness of God's presence with him.

The following evening we were invited to have dinner with my niece and family. As we were seated around the table, we all joined hands and prayed for a special anointing and healing for Roger. I felt a warm glow and deep assurance that God was indeed intervening in this new crisis. I believed that he would be healed of pneumocystis, *not of AIDS.*

We decided to take the southern route home and drive through scenic Brown County, Indiana. Color splashed through the trees as if tossed by a madcap wastrel—yellows, golds, red, and browns, shining like polished silk against the blur of purple hills. We were awed as we drove throughout the parks and mountain ranges. The bright blue sky in the warm October sun made the landscape breathtaking. God was proclaiming his glory and confirming to us his love and faithfulness!

There was the quiet assurance that he indeed was our loving heavenly Father who was doing all things well, and we could joyfully entrust the care of our son and all our family into his keeping.

Truly he is Lord!

10

Faithful Friends

Telephone calls from California became even more frequent. It seemed that with each call came a new concern for another disease, a different infection, more suffering. Could I advise concerning proper diet for gastrointestinal disease, amoebic dysentery, nausea, and vomiting? The ulcerated areas in his mouth and throat took away desire and taste for food. What kind of high-caloric drinks and food were most helpful? As I was a trained nurse, he trusted my judgment.

The next time it may have been a cry for help in treating hemorrhoids and/or constipation, severe headaches, massive scaling skin condition and psoriasis, night sweats, and coughing. Because of the neuropathy, he was experiencing pain just by touching or repositioning.

Annie, who lived in an apartment directly above his, had stairway access to his dining room area and had faithfully assisted him with meals, bathing, cleaning, shopping, and other needs. This care had become increasingly demanding.

Unlike many other people with AIDS, Roger did not have a lover to assist with his care. In reading through his journals we learned that he felt much rejection in not being suitable for a companion. From his Bali journal he wrote:

I believe that the fact that no one at home is ever interested in me sexually makes me enjoy the attention I'm getting. Probably I'm giving off mixed vibes because it's such a switch, and I like being noticed even though I'm not interested in following through on anything. Today I feel very confused and disoriented. I can't figure out what's happening with me. So many emotions. I want to cry and can't. I feel very lonely, sad, and depressed. I feel frail and helpless, like I need desperately to be held and comforted. I can't believe how rejected I feel or why this is coming up. Tonight I don't even want to see any friends for dinner and I certainly don't want to be alone. Feel too frail and brittle to engage in interaction with the Balinese. Afraid of being hurt as I was the other night when I was open and vulnerable. Anger, anger, anger. Feel like I don't even want to be here anymore, and I certainly don't want to go home. Feeling such loneliness and despair in the midst of all this beauty is horrible. Very, very heavy.

Even though Roger was denied a romantic relationship, he developed some deep friendships. He had a lasting relationship with Rosemary whom he learned to know in college. It was largely because of her that he moved to California. She said he was her "soul-mate." She remained his faithful friend throughout his illness and assisted with his care on her time off from her job. He kept his Day-Timer current with her working hours and time off and looked forward to her visits.

Roger was a person given to orderliness and detail. As his illness progressed, it became increasingly difficult for him to manage his business affairs. Ted, a friend he came to appreciate, assisted him with this detail and paid daily visits. Their shared love for music brought them together. Often after rehearsals of the Gay Men's Chorus, they were together for times of fun and relaxation. They enjoyed opera and ballet in the famous Opera House.

Roger's illness brought increasing demands on these special people; they were experiencing burnout. Ted had seen far too many of his friends die from this horrible disease and the possibility of his own susceptibility was always with him.

Annie, in early retirement from her employment with the airlines, had made previous plans to spend the next year in Bali. The problem of knowing how he could survive without the aid of these care-givers confronted him.

It was eight o'clock one evening in November when we received another call from San Francisco.

"Mom, I need you so badly!" The sobbing at the other end of the line indicated his desperation. "Can you come?"

I didn't hesitate. "Yes, of course. What is going on with you right now?" I probed.

"I can't tell you how bad it is. Could you come as early as tomorrow?"

Such fear and anxiety I had not heard before. His bitter sobbing prevented him from giving details.

"I need you. . . . Please come!" His voice broke with tears.

It was my turn to cry. Marvin was not at home. Banks and travel agencies were already closed by then.

Comforting verses of Scripture streamed into my mind as I prayed for guidance:

"God is our refuge and strength, An ever-present help in trouble" (Psalm 46:1).

I knew the Lord would not fail me, for he is faithful.

I put feet to my faith and started packing when Marvin came home. He was personally acquainted with the manager of the travel agency and called her at home. An hour and a half later she personally delivered our plane tickets to our home. We would leave the Wichita airport at seven in the morning. Talk about miracles! We knew for certain that God had intervened in our behalf.

Sheryl and Leo agreed to get up at four in the morning, drive an extra 60 miles, and take us to the airport. What comfort to know that our family stood by us.

Thoughts and emotions ran rampant across our minds as we boarded the plane:

Is Roger dying soon? . . . What can we do about his care? . . . The demands are too much for his friends. Physically and emotionally it's impossible to continue as it is now. . . .

In a telephone conversation a week ago, I had asked him about the possibility of securing hospice care. He had applied and was on a long waiting list. There was not enough personnel for the demands, they said. There were 32 critical persons ahead of him. We could not bring him home. How could he be so far away and need us so much? A thousand questions bounced from our lips as we flew above the big white cauliflower clouds.

And the really big question cropped up: *Was he really ready to die?*

He had committed his life to Christ when he was 12, but in his subsequent search for identity he had lost touch with his faith. Was his chosen lifestyle against God's will? In a previous conversation he had said he was ready to die. Had he truly repented? I remembered his mention of "guilt" during our first visit. Still, he hadn't been completely open to discussion of spiritual matters.

Since then he'd had time to think, although emotional pain and apprehension as well as physical agony had clearly confused him. Had he groped his way back to God?

The complexity of the whole situation seemed more than I could handle. Were it not for the undergirding of God's everlasting arms, I would have gone to pieces. Marvin will be able to figure out something, I assured myself. I could depend on him. I reasoned that men tend to be more rational and their thinking more calculated and systematic. They may not get as emotionally involved, but this was our only son. It was different. Marvin too was emotionally involved. Well, I had to be strong for him—so we were strong for each other.

We decided to avoid the confusion and congestion of the San Francisco airport and schedule to Oakland, rent a car, and drive an extra hour. The hectic traffic kept our minds focused on driving and, with God's help, we arrived at Roger's apartment safely.

I was hardly prepared for the suffering that greeted us when we walked in.

"Oh, I'm so glad to see you!" The weak hug and long embrace were so genuine. Tears filled my eyes as my heart reached out in a shared suffering that only a mother-heart can know.

The clutter completely hid the coffee table and bedside stand: bottles, medications, ointments, glasses of juice and water amidst dishes of dried fruits, nuts, and candy. The crumbs and scales from his skin disorder so covered the navy oriental rug that the pattern was hardly visible. It was stifling hot, yet he was covered with blankets and afghans, still struggling to keep warm.

We had scarcely exchanged greetings from family and friends when he suddenly announced his need for help to the bathroom. With great effort I assisted him, then left until he was ready to return.

Suddenly we heard a chilling scream of pain. "Mom, Please come and help me. . . !" I rushed to his side. Tears were rolling down his cheeks as I cradled his head in my hands and held him close.

"Please pray that it won't hurt so bad. Please God, I can't stand it" he sobbed.

I didn't hesitate a second. "Please, Father, you who are all-powerful and able to do even more than we can ask, come and be with us here right now. Give comfort and healing in body and spirit. Give us wisdom to know how to deal with this dreadful affliction. Please, give immediate relief from this awful pain!"

The severe pain subsided and I helped Roger back to bed. I thought a back rub might help him relax, and I could feel the tenseness ease as I began to massage him gently. Dad comforted him by rubbing his feet: he loved his dad's touch, and the foot rubbing became quite a ritual.

I took inventory of all his medications. Small wonder he was having trouble. I decided to talk to his primary physician.

With evening approaching we thought it best to make reservations for a motel. On the way from the airport Marvin had spotted one high on a ridge above Highway 101, away from heavy traffic. I had quickly jotted down the name and location. That motel became our haven for this and six following visits. It was reasonably priced and overlooked the bay in a quiet setting. We thanked God many times for showing it to us. It offered laundry services and a convenient coffee shop open 24 hours a day.

It was the Tuesday before Thanksgiving Day. I wanted it to be memorable since it no doubt would be the last one we would spend with Roger. As I began discussing it with him, he told me that all plans had been made to have eight of his close friends share the day with him in his home in traditional style. Each one was contributing something for the dinner: turkey and dressing, mashed potatoes, gravy, cranberry salad, pumpkin pie, plus other goodies. One of the fellows even made yeast rolls and bread from scratch. Roger had one request to make the menu complete: I was to make his favorite butterscotch pudding. I need not concern myself with any of the other food preparation, he added.

I was more concerned about his care and tolerance for the day than the food. He knew it would be his last Thanksgiving on earth and he wanted it to be very special. He wanted a fire in the fireplace and candles burning on his mantel. I wondered what effect all the extras would have on his ability to cope. but if he wanted it, we would try to make it happen.

Dinner was scheduled for 2:00 p.m. It was a bit of a trick to handle all the extras in his tiny kitchen. Annie offered her oven for needed space. All was ready at the scheduled time. Ted became host and invited everyone to gather around Roger's bed.

"This is a special day. It is Thanksgiving Day. We do have things to be thankful for. We are all here and have each other." Ted spoke with deep emotion. "Let's all take each other's hands and bow our heads in silent prayer."

Roger reached up his hands to make the circle complete. All eyes were misty as he spoke the *amen.* God knows the prayers that were in every heart that day. An attempt was made to make the meal a cheerful time and one of celebration, and Marvin and I struggled to choke down our dinner. To everyone there, it was "family" and traditional, in keeping with the usual holiday celebration.

We put a sampling of everything on Roger's plate, but he could eat very little. After dinner he wanted so much to join the others in the living room. There was laughter, storytelling, snacking, and listening to the crackling fire in the grate. We helped him out of bed and to the living room, but in a few minutes he had to return to his bed. It was so sad that he couldn't join in the celebration. The grim reality was that he could never fully enjoy any meaningful activity anymore. To share in that suffering is also difficult, even though one cannot *really* share it.

"You may be sad because you are losing me, but I am losing *all* of you!" Roger said in a wistful voice.

I wanted so much to make things better.

The next day I discussed his condition with his doctor, who offered to send out the hospice nurse for an evaluation to determine Roger's eligibility for hospice care. If his condition warranted it, he might have priority admittance. We made an appointment for the next afternoon.

We met Peggy and instantly loved her. She was a very warm, caring person. It was while she was there that Roger experienced one of his very severe pain attacks. I believe that was allowed by divine Providence! She said that he qualified for immediate admittance—and for a full eight hours daily with a professional care-giver. What wonderful news! She didn't know how he could get along at night without assistance, but he had been surviving with the help of his friends until late into the night. Hospice would not be able to provide more than eight hours.

It was decided that his nurse would work a split shift: 9:00 a.m. to 1:00 p.m. and from 4:00 p.m. to 8:00 p.m. with volunteers assisting in the hours between. How could we thank God enough for such an outpouring of love? He truly does not forsake his own.

The next few days were busy getting everything set up. A visit from the social worker entailed many details, and legal papers had to be signed. Time was running out; we needed to return home. Several days before we left we met Derek, his nurse. He was a very gentle, caring person. Roger liked him immediately, and that was important.

Annie, who had cared for him all these months just

because she loved him, was leaving for Bali. It was time to say good-bye. Her furniture and personal possessions had to be moved into storage. What a sad day! They knew it was a last farewell, and they needed some time alone. We went to our motel room for a rest. She seemed to us a long-time friend. She had so freely shared her love for Roger. With tears of affirmation for her kindness and a fond embrace we told her good-bye.

"Please keep in touch. I have come to love you too," she told us huskily.

On the wall of the foot of Roger's bed hung a large oil painting that he had brought from Bali. Attached to the lower frame was a light which showed up the beautiful Indonesian landscape. He spent many hours meditating as he viewed that picture, remembering its beauty and the peace he experienced while visiting there. It would help bridge the space between him and Annie while she was in that setting, and he would not forget her.

By now we had his medications regulated and he was more comfortable. Hospice care was set up and in motion. His noon and evening meals were prepared and delivered by Open Hands. Our tickets scheduled us to leave in the morning.

"You needn't come this evening," Roger told Derek." I'll spend it with my folks."

I promised to do his treatments and get him ready for the night before we left.

The intimate touch of rubbing his back brought special joy, and it gave us time to talk.

"Are you afraid?" I asked as I stroked his back gently.

"No, not anymore," he said quietly.

"Are you prepared to die?"

"Yes. It's okay." After a pause he asked, "Did you think I was going to hell because I am gay?"

I drew a sharp breath. "No, not because you are gay.

There are a lot of things I don't understand about that. I've tried to understand the struggle for identity you've had; the rejection you have felt at times; and the orientation, comfort, and love you feel for the same sex. What I don't understand is the need for sexual intercourse and related activities. I accept the biblical standard that sex is to be reserved for marriage between man and woman. For me, the principle outside of marriage is the same, be it heterosexual, bisexual, or homosexual. I know that innate desire is something that is difficult to deal with, and temptation is not the same for everyone. We *all* have temptation, and we all need to learn how to deal with it."

"I understand," he said.

I waited for further dialogue, but he continued on another thought.

"Sometimes at night I think about heaven. I think about Grandma."

"What do you think heaven will be like?" I prodded.

"Something like Bali." Again he related the beauty, harmony, and peace he experienced there. It must have made a tremendous impression on him, I thought.

"Do you still believe that Jesus died to save us and we have to believe in him in order to get to heaven?" he asked very thoughtfully.

"Yes, I do. Jesus said, 'I am the way, the truth, and the life: no man cometh unto the Father, but by me.' One of the first verses you ever learned, says so: 'Whosoever believeth in *him* should not perish, but have everlasting life.' I believe that Jesus came and gave his life for us. He was willing to die for my sins, and by that act he gave me the hope of eternal life" (John 14:6; 3:16, KJV).

Roger looked off into the distance and said, "Boy, that's really heavy. One of my very best friends is a Jew. There has never been a nicer person. She is just a jewel.

I can't believe she couldn't go to heaven."

A fragile silence hung between us, as though the subject was closed.

After a long pause, his face flushed, his eyes glassy, he went on: "Well, you have to go, I guess. I wish you didn't have to leave. Thank you so much for coming and for all you did for me. I don't know what I'd do without you." His voice sounded so miserable and weary.

Oh, how I hated to say good-bye to my son! He reached his arms up for a hug.

"I love you, Mom," he said huskily.

"I love you too, so very much. If I don't see you again, I'll meet you in heaven," I said, my lips shaking. With tear-filled eyes I walked away.

It was Marvin's turn.

"I'm sorry that I wasn't the dad I should have been," Marvin began, then choked up.

With his arms around Dad, Roger said, "Please, Dad, don't. We said we would forget the past and we don't say such things. Everything is okay."

Marvin nodded. "See you in heaven if not before."

The lights were turned low, fresh drink and juice by his medications with schedule cards, the telephone cradled on his bed, urinal nearby, and extra covers at the foot of the bed. Roger looked around carefully to see that all was in place.

With a wave of our hands, we locked his door and entrusted him to the care of our heavenly Father.

In the gateway between two doors, my strength seemed to drain from me, and I sagged against the wall.

"I'm okay," I mumbled heavily. I tried to make myself believe it. I shivered in the chilly night, and we drove away in silence. There were no words to express our sorrow. To have each other was enough for now.

11

Christmas

Christmas—the word itself floods my mind with all kinds of warm, nostalgic thoughts and happenings. The festive atmosphere, busy shoppers, music and merriment everywhere, the goodies, parties, dinners, programs, decorating, and plans for family dinners, with never enough days in the December calendar.

There were plans for dinner with our family, with the in-laws, and with extended family on both sides. There were dinners and parties with employer/employees. Somewhere we would squeeze in time for the church Christmas program, school program, college concerts, and on and on! I had always enjoyed the season. Decorating the house and making all the extra goodies was fun. *Peppernuts*—those dainty dime-sized morsels were a *must* even though it took what seemed like forever to cut those delectable tiny cookies.

Christmas this year (1985) would be different. We wanted to spend the day with Roger as we would probably never have another one with him. Even the thought made me sad. But it wasn't fair to deny our girls and families the celebration. They couldn't go to California, and Roger was not able to come home. It was decided that we would spend Christmas Day at home with Janene and Bob, Sheryl and Leo, and grandchildren

Denise and Craig. The following day we would fly to San Francisco for our Christmas with Roger.

This year I had little interest in the usual activities. Somehow I couldn't make sense or become excited about the joyous season. Sheryl and Janene persuaded me to put up a Christmas tree. I baked peppernuts because Roger was so fond of them and by now it was a tradition with us.

The programs that I always enjoyed so much left me with a big lump in my throat. Would there ever be days when we could be free of all this heaviness? It would never be the same again. With renewed determination, I decided to live only one day at a time; and I knew I had the promise for that.

With plans for Christmas dinner finalized, we had our tickets for an early morning flight to San Francisco the day after Christmas. Roger was very eager for our visit. He had many concerns about making a will, someone to take care of all his business, keeping volunteers and care-givers coming regularly, and just taking care of his basic needs. In his daily calls we tried to assure him that we would help to put things in order when we arrived.

There were times when he called because he felt so lonely and almost abandoned by his friends. Little did he know how demanding his care had become; some of his loyal friends were not able to cope with the situation. He had a right to his feelings, and I helped him to think through what was happening.

Christmas morning dawned crisp and clear. Our family ate breakfast together. As Marvin was helping me with dinner preparations, the doorbell rang; he answered it and came back with a vase of twelve long-stemmed red roses. "To all my family. I love you—Roger," the card said. There were no words as we faced each other, only tears. And then we continued our day in a daze.

It has been our tradition to eat dinner, clean up and wash dishes, then retire to the living room for devotions. Sometimes we do some responsive readings or a variety of things, but always Marvin reads the Christmas story and leads in prayer. Sometimes we join in petitions for different things. This morning we had some concern as to how we were going to be able to follow through. Our hearts were too full of emotion. As had become a daily need, we again asked for strength and guidance. We have come to know that God's provisions are abundant.

We called Roger following dinner, and all took turns wishing him a merry Christmas and acknowledged our love for him and thanked him for the lovely remembrance of roses. Marvin led the devotions, read the Christmas story, and turned it over to Leo to finalize that time. The gift exchange followed. Denise passed out the gifts. Roger's were to stay under the tree until they could be included in our packing. What gifts could we select for him? He was already thinking of giving up his things. He couldn't read, couldn't be up to do anything, and he had sufficient linens and clothes. What could symbolize our love?

Craig had a clever idea which proved to be a prized gift in the days and weeks that followed. He went downstairs to Grandpa's workshop. With the jigsaw he cut a piece of wood and then crafted words on it:

We ♥
You, Roger.

He painted the heart red and varnished the wood. It was a perfect gift. It was to become his constant companion, carried with him to the hospital and from the lab to Xray to wherever he was wheeled. He said it gave him courage.

Leo and Sheryl spent the night with us so they could take us to the airport early the next morning. They also promised to take down the Christmas tree and all the decorations.

Early morning, after a few hours of sleep, we were on our way to the airport. As a family we took turns encouraging one another. Encouragement is awesome. It has the magnetic power to draw us helpless humans to the God of hope, the one whose name is Wonderful Counselor, Mighty God, Prince of Peace. The one who is above all others!

Questions tumbled all over each other: How much longer will Roger be given life? . . . How much more must he suffer? . . . Why was he allowed to become victim to this dreadful, always fatal disease? The more we gave in to our feelings, the more questions continued to surface.

Already there were some signs of brain impairment. Roger found it difficult to remember details and telephone numbers. It was hard to process what was necessary to address his needs. He wrote with great difficulty, for he could not control pen or pencil. How could we best give him comfort and care?

All kinds of negative thoughts surfaced.

Did I lack obedience or was I not faithful? Tears of repentance and searching continued over and over. I found comfort in Scripture.

> My flesh and my heart may fail,
>   but God is the strength of my heart and my portion
> forever. . . .
>   I have made the Sovereign Lord my refuge. (Psalm 73:26, 26)

Soon we were on the plane. We lifted off in an overcast sky and soared above to a huge sea of billowy white fluff. An enormous red sun shone on the eastern horizon. It was a beautiful sight. Peace came from the calm assurance that we were again in the arms of the heavenly Father, going on a mission of love.

One o'clock found us ringing our code at Roger's door. We unlocked the door and were eagerly greeted by his smiling face.

"I'm so glad to see you. Merry Christmas!" he cried, followed by a long, warm embrace. My cheek against his very warm one confirmed his elevated temperature. His eyes appeared gaunt and sad, but his smile was as wide as usual. The room was stifling hot, yet the bed covers were piled high.

"Hello there," Marvin boomed. "We made it in record time. I'm beginning to feel like a California-style driver!" He always had cheer in his voice and could be depended on to make things better. He was a tower of strength and I was so thankful for him.

"Merry Christmas to you, Roger. We love you," I added. In the corner of his bedroom stood a beautiful eight-foot tall arrowhead plant, entwined with lights, some white doves, and a few ribbons to make it appear festive, like a Christmas tree. Isn't it a lovely thing someone has done? I thought. On his coffee table were the usual—fruit, nuts, and candy. In the kitchen and in the refrigerator were numerous gift boxes of fruits, nuts, and sweets that friends had brought in keeping with the spirit of Christmas.

Volunteers from the Shanti organization had planned a special Christmas party for AIDS patients. In our daily phone conversations, Roger told us he had wanted so much to go and made plans for one of the volunteers to take him. It was an event he could anticipate. The hospice nurse dressed him for the party. How eager he was for this special event where he could meet other fellows who were ill as he was, and also a host of support persons.

The volunteer picked him up as planned and took him to the party. It was a gala affair with balloons, treats, gifts, music, and many happy faces. His weakened condition had left him with little energy and few coping skills in this crowd, so his stay was short and he needed a bed. He had to come home, but with a good memory of the holiday spirit. How very fatigued he could become with the least exertion. To be remembered was enough.

There were stacks of cards and good wishes from friends near and far. I was so thankful that he had not been forgotten. He urged us to go through the mail and read all the encouraging letters and notes from family, friends, and loved ones. I was grateful for all the cheerful messages he had received.

His Day-Timer was always on his bed next to his telephone with the hospice emergency number on the cradle and a large yellow scratch pad close by. He could try to scribble notes and reminders, but they were barely legible. On the pad he had written a message, which I tried to read:

> It's a _____ for all of us with AIDS but an opportunity to heal out our lives and to grow spiritually. An opportunity for unity and love. We can survive by going together and believing in ourselves. Love yourself and love your brothers who are dying. We will all be together one day.

Who was the intended recipient of this message? I wondered. I found it much later as we went through his papers.

I believe he had come to the "acceptance" phase of his illness. He had previously experienced the various stages of dying, as does any other patient, regardless of the diagnosis. He had gone through a period of denial, anger, depression, and probably bargaining, and now he freely spoke of dying. It made it much easier.

Late afternoon Marvin and I went to the supermarket shopping for the makings of a Christmas dinner: chicken to fry, potatoes to mash, with cream gravy, corn, fresh vegetables for salad, and ingredients for butterscotch pudding. I chose carrot-bran muffins from the Honey Bakery instead of baking bread. It was one of his favorite foods anyway. Thirty minutes in my kitchen was equal, in cooking accomplished, to two hours in his tiny, inadequate one.

Being an organized person, Roger wanted to recap the agenda for the week. That night we reviewed and projected. He knew where he needed help. His first concern was to write his will and detail disposition of belongings. He needed a power of attorney and a durable power of attorney for health care. He wanted a systematic schedule of his care-givers, day and night. He also had concerns about his medical bills.

It all seemed so overwhelming. One's mind does not conceive of making plans for the final days for a *child.* Somehow, stored back in one's mind, one has an occasional thought of the possibility of a spouse being separated by death. It's not a possibility you entertain for long, but it is a fact. You never expect to lose a child first.

Numerous friends came as I was preparing our Christmas meal. My appetite had fled, but I set a company dinner table with a Swedish candelabra centerpiece I had brought for his Christmas gift. The seven candles were lit and Marvin prayed:

> Dear Lord, this is a very special day. We're so thankful that Jesus came, that he suffered and died for us, and

that by believing in him we have eternal life and through the resurrection we too will live beyond this life with you forever. We pray for comfort for Roger, relief from pain and anxious care. Just hold him in your arms today and give him your peace. Thank you for providing for our needs and for this special meal we can have together. In the precious name of Jesus, we pray. Amen.

"Oh, what a lovely dinner," Roger burst out. "I love the candles!"

As we passed the food, I noticed that he had filled his plate.

"Fried chicken and everything!" he exclaimed.

I put a few things on my plate, but didn't know if I could choke it down.

"Aren't you going to eat, Mom?" he asked with concern.

"I'm eating . . . I'm just not hungry," I parried. I noticed Marvin's plate looked rather skimpy, too.

Roger was always concerned with good nutrition and good health habits. Staying fit had been one of his trademarks before his illness.

After a few bites, I noticed that he was looking at his plate rather than eating. His appetite was gone, but he had always force-fed himself.

"It is so good but I just can't eat anymore," he said with a wry smile. He was noticeably tired. Usually he could sit long enough to finish a meal, then he would fall into bed totally exhausted and cover up so he could stop shivering.

So this was our Christmas dinner! The thought was like a bitter taste in my mouth.

Friends were in and out until 9:30 that night. Most brought flowers; he always had fresh flowers.

Evening cares followed. As I gave him his treatments, medication, and back rub, we reflected on past Christmases, the serenity of home and family. It all had special meaning for him, and he told us that we had been such great parents. We were humbly grateful for this response. He spoke of Grandma Hostetler. She had been very precious to him and he still felt sad that he could not attend her memorial service. She was very proud of all her grandchildren, and she prayed for each consistantly. She was always ready with little treats when they stopped in. She had cared for herself and was very alert until she died of a heart attack at the age of 96. He said he expected to see her, as she was waiting for him in heaven! His words were such a comfort to us.

We tucked him in, put an additional heater by his bed, replenished juice and water, laid out medications for nighttime, placed urinal on the bed, checked phone for dial tone, and then turned the lights low. I wrapped him in my arms for a good-night kiss and was thankful for the gift of life another day. I claimed the promise that the Lord is watching over us day and night (Psalm 121:3-8).

"If you need us in the night, our motel number is on your phone," Marvin said. "Please call us. We'll look forward to seeing you in the morning."

We told him good-night, locked the door, and headed for our motel. As we joined hundreds of cars on the freeway, I broke our silence.

"The world just goes on as though nothing has happened!"

No, it doesn't stop for us . . . .

12

Last Will
and Testament

Hospice personnel were in charge of Roger's total care. There were eight hours of paid professional care and numerous volunteers who also gave care. Assisting were volunteers from the Shanti organization who worked under contract and gave free services to those in need of aid and support. "Shanti" is a Sanskrit word meaning "inner peace." The Shanti Project logo is an eclipse, a circle within a square. The circle represents the inner world of the mind; the square portrays the solid reality of earth and body. United, they indicate the wholeness of the human being.

> This logo symbolizes the passage from light to darkness and return to light. For Shanti Project, it represents the changes brought about by illness and death, the darkness that can fall upon people experiencing these events, and the light that can follow in the wake of helpers who bring love and caring.*

Staffing was scheduled so that someone was there all but a few hours in the afternoon. The hospice registered nurse coordinator assumed responsibility for keeping

---

* From *Eclipse*, The Shanti Project Newsletter, Winter 1986.

charts current and medicine and supplies on hand. She made scheduled visits for evaluation and need, working in cooperation with the social worker, who also regularly visited Roger. They had so much love to give.

What would it feel like to know that all your patients were going to die, I wondered?

"We experience a lot of grieving," Peggy, the nurse, said soberly. "We become very attached to our patients, and they become as family. Most of our patients are rejected by families, who have nothing to do with their sons or daughters after they have been diagnosed with AIDS. People they have come to know become substitute family."

No wonder these care-givers grieve for those they have come to love.

"We are very surprised that you came," Peggy told us when we met. "We seldom see families who care enough to visit their sick children. But we're so glad you've come!"

The information was mind-boggling to me. How could parents *not* come? How could we *not* love our own flesh and blood? And the call to love is not just for parents:

> Love is patient, love is kind. It does not envy, it does not boast, it is not proud. It is not rude, it is not self-seeking, it is not easily angered, it keeps no record of wrongs. . . . It always protects, always trusts, always hopes, always perseveres. Love never fails. (from 1 Corinthians 13:4-8)

Love *never* fails. . . . I believe it! It breaks down walls, builds bridges, mends broken relationships. What does one have to lose? It broke my heart to think of the many suffering alienation. How thankful I was for these dear volunteers who gave countless hours of their time and love to Roger—because they cared! What a ministry they had. We came to love them very much.

The social worker had told Roger that a will can be legal and valid in court when a given form is used and handwritten. He had asked for a sample, which she brought. How much could it be abbreviated? Basically it need only state how he wanted his property and belongings dispersed, and by whom. He wanted his belongings to go to friends and family, and asked me to make a list of what we would like. That was difficult to think about.

"I want you to be responsible for giving certain things to specified persons," he told us. Of course, we assured him that we would do the best we could to carry out his wishes.

My concern was how he was gong to write *anything* in longhand. His hands shook so badly and it was difficult for him to hold a pen. I took the sample document, paper, and pen and sat down at the dining table. Peggy sat across from me, reviewing his chart and setting up his weekly medicine dispenser.

"How can you be so strong?" she asked, eying me, her brow furrowing. "I marvel as I watch you."

I shook my head and sighed. "I have to rely on the Lord, who gives me strength. It's very difficult." That was all I could say. Both of our eyes blurred as we continued our duties.

I prayed for wisdom and guidance as I wrote a sample, stating it as nearly as possible to Roger's request:

> I, Roger Oliver Hostetler, residing in San Francisco, California, declare this to be my first will. I leave all my possessions, earnings, insurance, and death benefits to my father, Marvin J. Hostetler of McPherson, Kansas. I designate my father, Marvin J. Hostetler, as executor of this my will to serve as such without bond. In the event that Marvin J. Hostetler is unable to serve as executor, I

nominate Helen Hostetler, my mother, to serve in his stead without bond.

January 1, 1986
Roger O. Hostetler

It was the most difficult assignment I had ever undertaken. For him, it took incredible effort. He worked with such diligence to make it legible, for it took so much effort for one word! He worked all afternoon to get it done. I was overwhelmed with his accomplishment. It was as though a big burden was lifted. Now he was relieved of the anxiety that surrounded the proper disposition of his earthly possessions.

Hospice personnel requested the need for a designated durable power of attorney for health care, should the need come in our absence. Someone was needed to make health-care decisions if for some reason he was unable to make the decisions for himself. By signing this document he was saying that he did not want life-sustaining treatment to be provided or continued if the burdens of the treatment outweighed the expected benefits. His agent would consider the need for relief of suffering, the quality of life, and the possible extension of his life in making decisions concerning life-sustaining treatment.

It wasn't easy to understand all that this implied. No one was eager for this assignment, for it carried so much responsibility. Rosemary, his longtime friend, seemed the logical agent and was his choice. She was reluctant to commit herself to such a grave task, but when we suggested Jan as an alternate to serve with her, she willingly consented. Jan had become very dear to him. Being a clinical psychologist, she had some helping skills, which greatly benefited Roger in handling his trials. She was a very sensitive, gifted person, and agreed to co-sign the document. Both hoped they would never need to exercise their power.

We were happy to see Roger at peace with these details. It was a new experience for all of us to deal with matters concerning death. One by one the "to do" list items were scratched off. He wanted a large calendar with pictures of beautiful flowers and a box by each date in which to jot down schedules of his care-givers. We finally found the kind of calendar he had in mind and placed it on the wall at the foot of his bed so he could see and plan ahead.

Was it chance that brought Doug to his door one cool, damp evening after work? With a bunch of flowers in his hands, he greeted Roger warmly. They soon discovered they know some of the same people. Doug was also a graduate of Goshen College, a year later than Roger, and a member of the San Francisco Mennonite Fellowship. Later I learned that I also knew his mother through college connections. As we reminisced about past events, I was certain God had sent Doug to be his ministering angel. Only God heard my inaudible thank-yous over and over! He was to become an outstanding care-giver for Roger's remaining days.

In a visit with the social worker we learned that an immediate decision needed to be made in assigning someone for his power of attorney and also someone designated as his primary care-giver. His three very close friends were not able to handle the assignment, and we needed to return home. What should we do? I remembered the words from Proverbs 4:11-12:

> I guide you in the way of wisdom and lead you along straight paths.
> When you walk, your steps will not be hampered;
> when you run, you will not stumble.

As we left our motel the next morning we believed that promise. We had learned to trust totally, implicitly, for the task was too big and awesome for us.

When we walked into Roger's apartment the next morning, he greeted us with a glint in his eyes. "Doug has offered to help me wherever I need him!" he said with a quiet joy.

"Praise the Lord!" I cried. Oh, how good God really is!

"He called just to visit," Roger went on. "I told him I needed someone as my power of attorney and also someone as my primary care-giver."

As we discussed the need for both, we reasoned that with paying of bills and taking care of insurance for health needs, Roger's business affairs presented an immediate need. He already had numerous care-givers and his basic needs were being met. We were relieved when Doug agreed to assume responsibilities for Roger's power of attorney. He was to become a vital link to the peace Roger experienced in his final hours.

Our very breath became an awareness of God's presence, which made life meaningful and full of promise and hope. It was the only way we could survive. Knowing Roger's friends loved him made it so much easier for us. The quality of the love they extended will always hold a special place in our hearts. It was spontaneous and unconditional.

The gift of life took on special meaning. One by one Roger's friends and acquaintances had become victims of this terrifying, fatal disease. Who would be next? Five employees from the Pacific Bell office in which he worked had already died. Among some of his friends there was a paranoia that required regular counseling and support groups. Fear of being rejected by their families was the most common concern. Over and over we heard stories of families who refused to allow their sons to return home, and who did not visit or have any communication with them. At a time when families were needed most, they failed to be available. Is this how the servant Jesus loved?

> Surely he took up our infirmities and carried our sorrow. . . . He was pierced for our transgressions, he was crushed for our iniquities. . . . and by his wounds we are healed. We *all* . . . have gone astray, each of us has turned to his own way; and the Lord has laid on him the iniquity of us all. (Isaiah 53:4-6)

My heart ached for them. How can we choose whom to love? The price was paid for all!

> Bob Russell wrote the following in an article, "Heroes and Heroines of Our Time," in *Eclipse* (Fall 1987):
>
> In Oct. '83 I attended a three-day workshop with Kübler-Ross for people with AIDS. It was at Wildwood. I bicycled there and back from San Francisco and became known as the *bicyclist with AIDS*. The experience I got from the workshop profoundly affected me, and I moved into a house with two other men with AIDS. We all appeared healthy, but within three months my first roommate had died. There was no will. Friends and family (born-again Christians from the Midwest) arrived, ransacking our home. Some of my possessions were taken as well. His family tried to set me down on my knees to be saved, renouncing my gayness and embracing their beliefs. That was fun.

I understood what Roger meant when he said, "Sometimes Christians can be so cruel." If only we could learn to model the life of Jesus and allow his love to touch others! My heart aches for all who find themselves caught in this dilemma. How much wisdom, patience, and understanding we need!

Once again we had completed the primary purpose of our coming and it was time to return home. Would there be yet another time? Roger had told his hospice nurse not to come that night because he wanted to be alone with us. We too wanted it to be a special occasion. When he was too tired to talk, we bathed him in silence, just touching him. As Marvin rubbed his feet, he found it very soothing. It was so good for Marvin to do something physically to bring Roger comfort. I gave him his treatments and medications and a last back rub.

"I don't think I'll be here very long anymore," he said after I was finished.

"Are you afraid of dying?" I asked. My breath caught in my throat.

"No, not anymore. I think some night I will just slip away. I will quit breathing and I'll find myself in heaven. It will be peaceful and beautiful, and will remind me of the Garden of Eden—and Bali. I'll be able to see Grandma. She's waiting for me, you know. Sometimes at night . . . I just sort of drift away into unconsciousness . . . seems like I quit breathing. Some night I think it will be like that and I'll just be gone," he ended in a husky whisper.

It was difficult to keep my emotions under some restraint. Swallowing hard I said, "I am so thankful that you are at peace. Do you remember when you accepted Jesus as your Savior?"

"Yes, I sure do. I'm so glad that I remember it well," he said quietly. "Christ forgave my sins."

"Then it's like going home to your heavenly Father, who is eager for you, just as we are when you come home to us," I added.

"I do wish I could live awhile longer, but I have no quality of life here anymore. I'm tormented with so much pain . . . and I know I can never get well. I'm just anxious to be at peace in a neat place and get it all over with. You are so strong, but I'm sorry for you." He turned his head away and blinked back his tears.

"It's all right with us, Roger dear. It's hard for us to see you suffer, and very hard to give you up, but it will be so much better for you. Thank you for the joys you have brought us. We'll remember them. Just to be able to acknowledge our love for one another is a treasure to keep in our hearts forever." My voice had dwindled almost to a whisper.

The hour was late. Our emotions and bodies were weary. Would there be another time? After each visit it was harder to leave. Might a miracle drug be discovered in time to save Roger's life? Only God knew.

With hugs and wet eyes we bid him farewell. The thought of locking him in his house all alone was almost more than we could bear.

Why, Lord? Why us? Dared I ask the question? I remembered Job's anguish and misery. I also recalled the words of the psalmist: "The sacrifices of God are a broken spirit; a broken and contrite heart, O God, you will not despise" (Psalm 51:17).

It was as though God rode in our car as we prepared to leave. He said, "No good things does he withhold from those whole walk is blameless. O Lord Almighty, blessed is the man who trusts in you" (Psalm 84:11-12).

I meditated and prayed silently:

I believe in you, Lord. I trust you. Thank you for the good you are going to bring out of this sorrow. . . .

13

A Plan for Transition

An usual we anticipated an early morning call from San Francisco. More and more frequently they were collect calls. Roger could no longer dial nor remember familiar phone numbers. Often we received a second call within several hours. Sometimes he had forgotten he had called; other times he just wanted to tell us that he loved us and wished he could be with us.

The AIDS virus had begun neurological impairment. Dementia had begun. Of all the numerous infections he had survived, this seemed the worst. It was so out of character for him: the short attention span, going from one topic to another in rapid succession, the memory loss, and numerous dysfunctions. He was fully aware of his inability to perform as usual, but he couldn't help himself.

One morning, upon answering the phone, I got the usual greeting: "Hi, Mom. I love you." His voice was very weak. It was difficult to understand him. "I want to talk to both of you. Can you get Dad on the line, too?"

Marvin was already on the other phone.

"I had a long talk with Peggy yesterday," Roger went on. "I'm tired and am suffering so much. I have no quality of living at all, and I know I can never get well. She said that if I give up I'd probably die very soon. She was nice to talk to, and said other patients who gave up died right away. I'm tired of fighting. Could . . . could I have your blessing to just give up? Would it be okay with both of you, Mom? Dad?"

Our voices husky, we both answered in the affirmative, sharing his desire to be free from suffering and disappointments.

"Thank you both," he said with a tired sigh. "I have one more request. I want to see you once more. Do you think Leo and Sheryl could come? I want so much to see you all before I die and I think it will be soon. Do you think you could come as soon as tomorrow?"

Tomorrow? Could they make such sudden plans? I wondered. Could we even get tickets so quickly? As always, special-fare tickets were out of the question. The next hour we made a number of phone calls, debating whether we should encourage Janene to go without Bob, as we knew he couldn't get away from his job. Marvin thought it would be emotionally quite hard for Janene. We called her and told her of our conversation with Roger and of our plans to go. She cried as usual and said she would not plan to go.

The following morning the four of us headed for the airport. If Roger's time was here to die, we hoped it was while we were there. It would mean a lot to have Leo and Sheryl's support. We called ahead for motel reservations at Bayside Motor Lodge, which had become a haven for us away from the roaring freeway traffic, and overlooking the bay. It was a quiet restful reprieve from the busy days packed full of decision-making and cares.

We picked up our rented car at Oakland airport and drove to our motel to sign in and leave our luggage. Upon arrival, there was a emergency message for Leo. He was to call his parents immediately. From the look on Leo's face as he talked, we knew it was serious. Someone must be seriously ill. Why did it have to be now? I wondered. The conversation ended, he dropped the telephone cradle with a thud. His face clouded as he said, "Daryl's had a stroke. He's in intensive care at Wesley Hospital in Wichita." Daryl was Leo's younger brother. How could a stroke happen to a 40-year-old?

A dark cloud hung over us as we drove to Roger's house. Every mile was a prayer. Discussions shifted from Daryl to Roger. Hadn't we suffered enough? What were we to learn from all this?

Roger was eagerly waiting for our doorbell code. He already knew approximately when to expect us. The hugs were genuine, but his arms were weak. As usual, he beamed as he greeted us. We exchanged greetings and spoke briefly of our flight and plans.

Looking around, he said, "Didn't Janene come? I so much wanted her to come, too. I wanted all of us to be together this last time." Tears of disappointment dampened his eyes.

"We can call her and maybe she can make arrangements to come," Dad said.

"Please do. I want to see her."

Janene had to get in touch with Bob, who was in northern Kansas, and make arrangements with him about her coming. After several calls, we decided to meet her at the Oakland airport the following noon. In the meantime we exchanged calls between Wichita and San Francisco. Daryl's condition had worsened and the prognosis was poor.

I was in the kitchen trying to cook supper. Three of Roger's friends were present. No one was very hungry, but eating at mealtime is the customary thing to do.

I stepped into the bedroom and found Roger sobbing. "I feel so bad about Daryl," he cried. "I feel so sorry for Leo and Sheryl too. How can you be so strong?"

"My strength is only in the Lord, Roger. It isn't always easy," I said.

One of Roger's friends came out and put his hand on my shoulder. "How can you stand up under all this?"

"I depend on the Lord. He gives me strength."

He looked at me in disbelief, and I continued. "Yes, he *really* does. He is my strength."

Shaking his head he said, "I'm glad he gives *you* strength."

"And I'm so thankful for him," I said.

The next day word came that Daryl was put on a respirator. Leo and Sheryl needed to return home. Janene had come in on a morning flight. Motel accommodations were adequate for her to share our room since we had two double beds and a single bed. We decided on a quick tour of points of interest in San Francisco for the next day. Janene would return with Leo and Sheryl on a late-night flight, so she would not have to travel back alone.

Fisherman's Wharf had lost its interest for me, but I was grateful that we could see it together. We drove out to the beach and from the Cliff House listened to the roar of the sea lions and watched the waves lap along the shore. Sea gulls soared and dived with a series of wild, lonely cries that knifed through me like a pain. In the distance we could see several ocean steamers or cargo ships. The Pacific was endless. The sea rolled forward with crashing waves that blurred against the horizon. It was truly awesome, majestic!

In late afternoon we came back to Roger's for our final evening together—his wish. We reminisced and shared our joys, our disappointments, even our dreams. We expressed joy at having us all there together and felt he was going to die in peace soon. Then it was time for Leo, Sheryl, and Janene to leave for the airport. We all were reluctant to go. With final hugs and tears we said good-bye.

In a cheery voice Leo said, "We'll see you in heaven!"

Roger nodded.

Dad and I said good-night and that we'd see him in the morning; we planned to stay a week. The hospice nurse would be there early for the treatments and bathing, so we would come later.

Sleep didn't come easy. I am not a morning person and can usually sleep well when it's time to get up, but in San Francisco it was different. I awakened with morning. Perhaps it was the beauty of the pink sunrise reflected in the waters of the bay. It was like a special gift to us.

Before Marvin and I went to see Roger in the morning, we took the opportunity to see more of San Francisco. One morning we went to the zoo; another time we visited the arboretum, the museum, and other points of interest in Golden Gate Park. We viewed the city from the Twin Peaks and drove to the Golden Gate Bridge. We were discovering beauty we hadn't seen. We enjoyed eating prawns at Louie's, a short distance from the Cliff House. The large windows above the cliff presented a full view of the ocean. How vast it was! Small wonder that Roger loved it so much.

I recalled how impressed he was with this beauty when he first moved to California. In a letter dated August 26, 1977, he wrote:

> It's really fine here and I just love living here so much. It is really the perfect place and situation for me right now. I look at it all sometimes and just get blown away at how happy and satisfied I am with my life right now. I have been realizing more and more how there is really nothing more that I could ask for.

I appreciate so much David, Joan, and Tom. It is so good for me to feel such a strong part of their family and to have my work situation tied in with them. Our working relationships are not always problem free, but there is an underlying intention with all of us to contribute to each other's lives and it makes handling hassles that come up much easier. It is really the first job situation I've had where I felt no separation between my life and the way that I happen to be earning my living at the time. . . .

Bonita and I had a really terrific time together after four years. She was probably my most special friend through all the Indiana years. It was great to be able to pick right up where we left off. I flew down to Lynn and Bob's for a weekend while she was down visiting them so we could all be together again. It was a really wonderful time, of course. One night we went to see the Hollywood Bowl and heard the Los Angeles Philharmonic perform a Beethoven festival. It was so beautiful, being outdoors in the amphitheater with a full moon, listening to the 5th Symphony! We had a picnic/feast. Quite fun. We went to Big Sur and San Francisco and all the other places to sight-see.

It is so exciting for me to be living my life from a new perspective and to recognize my expansion. I sometimes get into lamenting over wasted time in my life. But I know that where I've been has all been necessary for me to be where I am now. My relationships are all so different for me, too. So many of them are really growing experiences. It feels so good.

Yes, it is comforting to recall the good years, to remember the meaningful and lasting relationships, and to forget the pain of the past. Those years were not all wasted. It is important to remind him of that. He needs affirmation, I decided.

Roger was concerned that his insurance and benefits

would terminate soon. It had been a year since he had worked full time. He had been selected from a final screening of 90 applicants for the position of service representative for priority accounts for Pacific Bell, a position which he held until his confinement. He asked Marvin whether he would be willing to visit with his supervisor and ask him to explain his benefits. Roger was afraid of not being able to grasp the explanation, since his mental capacities seemed dull at times. Marvin agreed and set up an appointment.

I will always be grateful for having been present to hear the supervisor relate to Roger and us what a valued employee he had been. He said he had devised an excellent plan in the use of the big rule-and-practice manual for additions and deletions. He said the plan would be in continued use with great efficiency. We heard him tell Roger that he was the most efficient employee, that he was greatly missed, and that no one sat at his desk. His voice was soft-spoken and clear, and he showed great compassion. His personality was warm and charming. We felt proud of Roger's achievements and glad we had met this gracious gentleman who affirmed Roger as an employee. Roger seemed pleased and thanked him.

"Your benefits will continue," the supervisor said.

When asked for how long, he added "Forever."

Roger sighed with relief and thanked him again.

"Please let me know if there is anything at all I can do for you," the supervisor said. With a warm handshake he left.

Once again it was time for us to return home. Roger had weathered his siege of attack. In AIDS, the patient may overcome one infection for a time, and then rally before the onslaught of the next. His condition remained about the same for a while. He was well cared for, his nurse was kind and compassionate, with a sensitive spirit, and volunteers assisted him.

Those who cared for him became very attached to him, for he had a sweet spirit and showed so much evidence of love. They said he was unusual and special. They stayed hours beyond their agreement. One thing puzzled them: how could Roger face death with such peace?

We were willing to release him to the Lord, if his time was up. Always in the back of my mind was the prophecy—that Roger would walk in obedience to the Lord. I believed it, for it was Spirit-breathed. How was it going to be totally fulfilled? And how long before the final victory?

My sister sent me a poem from *A Collection of Poems*, by Helen Steiner Rice, entitled "Before You Can Dry Another's Tears—You Too Must Weep." The message of the poem struck me, especially as summed up in its closing lines:

> God enters the heart that is broken with sorrow
> And he opens the door to a Brighter Tomorrow,
> For only through tears can we recognize
> The suffering that lies in another's eyes.

14

A Night of Celebration

In a telephone conversation a few days after our return home, Roger informed us of his desire for having a going-away party with his friends. He wanted his friends to know why he could die in peace. He would have it catered with a variety of delicacies, pastries, and goodies. He would have flowers, long-stemmed white roses (his favorite flower), and invite all his close friends, approximately forty.

He wanted fire in the fireplace and candles burning in holders. He would invite Randy, his hospice massage therapist, to have a session with him at the close of the festive part. Perhaps God would choose to take him at such a time.

He said we should pray for his release. He'd already called friends in far-off places, asking them to pray that he could die and go to heaven right there in the presence of his beloved friends. He also asked us to call our friends and extended family and agree together that God would take him home. With such eagerness and anticipation he planned it all in detail. His physical symptoms seemed to subside as he talked about plans.

Randy wrote about his relationship with Roger and about that going-away party:

The assignment has been made. "It's a good match," the volunteer coordinator said, as he gave me background and information. The new one was dying, of course, just like those before him. Nothing unusual. The list of symptoms was shocking and somehow comfortably familiar at the same time. "Reduced motor function, weight loss, pneumocyoistis, herpes, psoriasis . . ." he began, and the list went on.

I made the call. The first contact felt like a one-sided blind date. I knew about Roger—his medical condition, his mental state, his contagion. What did he get? A phone call from some stranger.

"Hello, is this Roger?"

"Yes." The reply was resigned and exhausted.

"I've been assigned to work with you by the hospice. My name is Randy. I'm one of the massage therapists."

We set up a session for the next evening. When I got to Roger's ground-floor apartment, the metal gate was unlocked and the front door beyond it stood open. What must it be like to lay open you life, to lose that sense of personal space? I squeezed the thoughts from my mind.

From the entry I could see Roger, lying in his bed. He had on a sweat shirt and sweat pants. They engulfed his boney frame. The eyes that looked up at me were child's eyes, unblinking and questioning.

The AIDS virus had done quite a job on him. Roger was close to six feet tall and weighed just about a hundred and twenty pounds. It must be scary living in a body you no longer recognize. After a lifetime of looking at yourself in the mirror, how hard it would be to alter the perception of your physical self.

For me, on that first visit, what I saw *was* Roger. There were no prior memories to buffer my impression. I would get to know the pre-AIDS Roger in time, though, through friends and photographs.

He treated me like a teacher does his students on the first day of classes. His domain had its rules and procedures. If I was going to fit in there was much for me to learn. By the end of the first session, he would have me well trained. I set up my portable massage table in the cramped bedroom, straddling the corner of the bed. He needed help onto the table and in undressing. Roger worked hard, doing as much for himself as possible. It was a slow process, but for him a very important one.

The massage started gently and became more specific as a subtle communication developed between us. I started on his back and worked my way down his arms. When I began to massage his hands they seemed to have a life of their own, moving like a cat tail moves. Each finger danced its own dance.

Over the months we became true friends. Fears were aired, disappointments vented, and hopes shared. Our lives became known to each other. Through Roger's stories, his friends became my friends.

One night before our last session, he said, "I'm going to have a going-away party. I want my friends to meet each other. I want to say good-bye." He asked if I would massage him the night of the party. I nodded.

The night arrived. When I got there, Roger was seated in a corner of the living room surrounded by a circle of people sitting on the floor. A fire was going and the rooms were filled with candles. They produced a rich, amber glow, turning white to yellow and red to orange. As I looked around, I noticed that he had put names on all of his possessions. They denoted who would get what he left behind.

One by one, people shared their feelings. Some spoke, others recited poetry, a woman sang. It was a safe place for us to communicate from our hearts. These were Roger's friends whom I had come to know through his stories. Now they were there in person. Roger was giving us his friendships.

When everyone had finished, a kind of satisfying silence filled the space. I asked him if he was ready for the massage. He smiled an acknowledgment and struggled up out of his seat. Then, without embarrassment, he undressed to his shorts and lay on the table.

I had never before worked on anyone with so many watching. It was not like at the hospitals where staff and visitors paraded in and out. This was more like a ritual.

One at a time, I motioned for his friends to come forward and begin to slowly rock Roger with their hands. Soon we were all there, our energy focused on him. Then in a determined voice he asked us to direct our thoughts toward his passing. We all did our best to help him in his transition.

Roger did not die that night. He wanted to let go so very badly. For him, it was the best way to go, surrounded by his loving and caring friends. But he didn't die. He would not have his perfect death. AIDS had taken control of his life; now it controlled his death.

We stayed a long time, until we finally helped him into bed. His disappointment affected each of us. We felt his helplessness.

Roger's story is not over. It continues at a slow pace,

sometimes enlightening, sometimes lonely and frustrating.

This is one story of many like it. There are thousands of individuals suffering not only from a debilitating, disfiguring disease but from total abandonment as well.

Most are not as fortunate as Roger. His friends and family did not reject him, afraid of a disease they don't understand. At least, we can be happy for this.

All evening and into the night our prayers and thoughts were for him. We prayed that if it was God's will, Roger's wish would be granted. He had suffered enough. Always there was the question: Was he really ready to die? Was there yet unfinished business? So many days and nights I had prayed, but always the burden was there. Why did I ask it over and over? It was my day of surrender! It occurred to me that I could just thank the Lord for what he was going to do and believe it to completion. It was as simple as that.

Audibly I said, "Lord, he is yours. He belongs to you. It is no longer my problem. Thank you for what you are going to do for him and with him." I had an unbelievable peace! I could rest in it. It was that profoundly simple!

The telephone had been silent all night. What would happen to his faith if his wish was not granted and he didn't die as he had wished? I need not wrestle with the thought.

15

One Last Wish

I began to feel panic every time the phone rang. What message will be next? I wondered. In the midst of all the business calls were always those well-wishes from friends and contacts from Roger three or four times a day. We suggested we would call every morning to avoid the high cost of collect calls, but Roger sometimes forgot. He just wanted to tell us that he loved us, and to update us on his latest concern. His voice had grown weaker and he tired very quickly; the calls were never very long. We were simply glad he wanted to talk to us.

The night of the party had gone by and we had no word from the West. As we wondered what might have taken place the night before, the telephone rang. It was Roger.

"Hello. Well, I'm still here." He sounded disappointed. "But it was a *wonderful* party! You wouldn't believe all the people who came! It was just great to be with everyone . . . and I think they all had a good time." He mentioned the goodies they had to eat.

"Could you eat and enjoy it too?" I asked.

"Well . . . ," he hedged, "not much. But they enjoyed it. Someone wrote a song for the occasion. We all sang it. It was so beautiful. I had a vision," he added eagerly. "And I saw Grandma! She stretched out her hands and said I should come." I could hear a faint sobbing on the other end.

"But I guess your time was not yet," I soothed.

He paused briefly and went on: "I meditated a lot during the night. I have one more request. I'd like to come home. Could I come?"

Come home? Roger—so ill: And he wanted to come: I didn't hesitate.

"Of course, we'd love to have you. but how could you manage to get here?"

"I'll fly. There are ways for sick people to fly. They have wheelchairs and attendants."

"Would you come alone?"

"Carol Ann may be able to come with me. If she can't, I can still make it. I'd like for you to have an elegant formal dinner, a real celebration. I'm going to borrow Jeff's tuxedo. Have the family dress in formal clothes," said Roger, always the planner.

What kind of elegant dinner did he have in mind? I asked.

"Fried chicken, mashed potatoes and gravy, butterscotch pudding, and—you know; like you do." Roger knew exactly what he wanted.

On the other phone Marvin asked about schedules and dates. Roger said he had thought it through carefully and had Jeff check for possible flights. Jeff would pack for him.

Roger was in earnest. He was really planning to come! I couldn't believe it. Was it a fantasy? I wondered. One of the half-baked ideas he'd had recently? I needed to be sure.

"Are you sure you can make it okay? Do you think your doctors would approve?" I asked. I still could hardly believe my ears.

He wanted to come immediately. "I think the Lord

healed me," he said quietly. "He didn't take me, so he must have healed me!"

Will surprises ever cease? A thousand thoughts tumbled through my mind. Could I even care for him? I wondered.

"Don't you think God could have healed me, Mom?" His voice held an urgency. I knew he wanted by confirmation.

Of course, I know that God has all power, but somehow I had trouble believing that Roger was healed. Was my mind playing tricks with me? Oh, Lord, give me wisdom, I prayed silently.

"What about hospice? Will they allow you to leave and pick you up when you return?" I said finally, needing to be practical. I urged him to make arrangements. Was that concern showing my lack of faith, or was it good common sense? It just seemed terribly complicated to me, almost too much to think about.

"Then it's okay if I come?" His tone was that of a child.

"We would love to have you, my dear." I meant every word.

Three telephone calls followed that day. Jeff was getting his ticket and definite arrangements were made for him to come in three days. He would include all his medications in his packing. I suggested he get a refill on his prescriptions because our local pharmacy might not stock them.

"Is there a crematory nearby in case I die while I'm home?" he asked. I was glad that we had previously arranged with our local mortician for future need and could answer some of his questions.

Am I physically able to give care twenty-four hours a day? The thought hammered at me.

"Can Sheryl and Janene help take care of me so that

it won't be so much for you, Mom?" he asked.

I knew that I *would* be able. I was so happy he wanted to come home. Maybe he will never be able to go back, I reasoned. Marvin was concerned that his care could be overwhelming. When I called to Sheryl and Janene they couldn't believe he was able to travel!

We prepared for a wonderful homecoming. We would give him our master bedroom, which had a bathroom and shower. It is also large enough for comfortable chairs plus other essentials. We purchased a shower chair to assist with his bathing. How would the community accept the presence of an AIDS patient in their midst? It didn't matter to us. He was our son. He deserved the best we could offer. We are willing to take the risk.

I was relieved when Dr. Claassen, our physician and a member of our church, agreed to assume responsibility for his care if needed.

Leo borrowed a van so that Roger would be comfortable and we'd all have room to meet his plane at the airport. Was Roger as excited about his visit as we were? we wondered. What if he forgot some of his medications? But he was in the care of our heavenly Father and that was enough. We would take each day at a time.

The plane was due at the airport in Wichita at 9:00 p.m. We arrived in plenty of time. Shortly after 8:30 the arrival time was posted as one hour late. Anxious thoughts crossed our minds. How could a sick, weary passenger wait an extra hour in a crowded airport in Denver? One hour later they posted another delay of an hour. We maintained our composure by meditating on Philippians 4:6-7, which called on us to have no anxiety, to pray, and to be kept by God's peace.

Two more delays were posted. The plane was now to arrive in Wichita at 1:00 a.m.! To ease our minds, Marvin asked about the condition of a passenger, Roger, giving the flight number with scheduled time of arrival. The computer message came back, saying he was in a wheelchair with an attendant and doing fine. The miracle of our communication system! The greater miracle was that once again God was proven faithful.

At long last the plane arrived. Passengers filed out until finally there was no more. We waited anxiously. Where was Roger? Marvin decided to walk down the ramp to the plane and find out what had happened. After what seemed like an eternity, we saw him pushing the wheelchair up the ramp with a smiling Roger in good spirits! There were greetings and hugs from us all. We picked up his bags and headed for home. Unbelievably, he said he'd enjoyed the extra time in Denver. He had called a college friend now living there, who came to the airport to see him. They'd had a great visit.

He had an attendant with him all the time, a wonderful service the airline provided. He had endured the long wait far better than we had.

We were glad to be home. Roger's head burned with fever and he needed his medication. I ransacked his bag for the bottles of pills and got him settled in bed. It was almost like a dream.

As I unloaded the suitcase filled with prescriptions and directions for his care, I realized the demands this schedule would hold, for it was important that the routine and medications should follow the hospice plan. But the joy of having him home would far exceed the demands, I reasoned.

After a tour of the house, Roger had expressed his joy to be with family. I tucked him into bed with his usual layers of blankets and afghans to keep warm.

Questions, however, continued to race through my

mind. Would our local hospital readily admit an AIDS patient, if necessary? Did our doctors have the expertise to care for one? We had done our homework. Although our local doctor had agreed to assume his care, he had never personally treated a patient with AIDS. We would live in faith hour by hour. We had learned it was the only way.

16

Time to Be Tender

Soon we shall all be the ones needing affirmation, encouragement, physical care, a touch of tenderness, and, most of all, love. We recall the timeworn counsel good Dr. Thomas Sydenham, the English Hippocrates (1624-1689), wrote to the professionals of his day:

It becomes every person who purposes to give himself to the care of others, seriously to consider the four following things: First, that he must one day give an account to the Supreme Judge of all the lives entrusted to his care. Second, that all his skill and knowledge and energy as they have been given him by God, so they should be exercised for his glory and the good of mankind, and not for mere gain or ambition. Third, and not more beautifully than truly, let him reflect that he has undertaken the care of no mean creature; for, in order that he may estimate the value, the greatness of the human race, the only begotten Son of God became himself a man, and thus ennobled it with his divine dignity, and far more than this, died to redeem it. And fourth, that the doctor being himself a mortal human being, should be diligent and tender in relieving his suffering patients, inasmuch as he himself must one day be a like-sufferer.*

---

* From *Christian Medical Society Journal*, 22:2, 1981, as quoted in Charles R. Swindoll, *Encourage Me* (Portland: Multnomah Press, 1982), page 55.

People who are hurting need to have more than an accurate diagnosis and a systematic program of therapy. They have a greater need to know that care-givers—be they doctors, dentists, therapists, nurses, attendants, parents, or family—are there because they do care. Roger was blessed to have this kind of support. Never have there been more loving physicians that those who attended him. Out of their busy, demanding schedules, they took the time to care for us, put their arms around us, weep with us, and tell us they were sorry. Was there any way they could help us? they asked. Would Roger perhaps miss the love and attention given him by numerous Shanti and hospice volunteers as well as professionals who helped him? Could our love and service give him enough and could we meet the increasing demands of his illness?

Though very weak, Roger decided he could walk in the house with a cane and the support of a chair, wall, or person. We tried to encourage him, yet also cautioned him against falling. The first days of his visit we reminisced a lot. We had so many fond memories to cherish. We also planned the elegant dinner he requested. To my surprise, he had brought along a tuxedo from his friend Jeff, whom he had learned to love so much. Jeff was a Shanti volunteer under contract as a practical aid person. He very ably took care of Roger's household needs, grocery shopping, laundry and ironing, house cleaning, dishwashing, numerous errands.

Roger grew very dependent on Jeff and eagerly anticipated his visits which became more and more often. We enjoyed talking to him and just being with him. Soon Roger recognized that Jeff gave of his time and energy out of love and he came to love Jeff very much. We loved Jeff too.

Shanti also provided a spiritual counselor named

Mark. He was assigned not to persuade him toward any creed or doctrine, but also to share his beliefs or questions and give him opportunity to process his thoughts on death and home. Mark, too, was special.

The dinner was planned and included last-minute preparations. This cook dressed a helpless guy with a tuxedo-cummerbund, starched and pleated shirt, bow tie and all. It had been many months since Roger had worn any kind of dress-up clothes. How he looked was very important when he was well. Now his hands trembled, his head was hot with fever, and the long-tailed satin-collared coat was far from keeping him warm. He was visibly shaking, but I couldn't hurry him. This really was important to him. He looked at himself in the mirror and gave a wary but genuine smile. I knew it was truly a time of celebration for him, and I wanted so much to please him. But I saw he had become very fatigued and feared he wouldn't be able to eat.

We poured the punch quickly and all sat down. Marvin suggested that we sing our prayer, "Praise God from Whom All Blessings Flow." The four-part harmony was beautiful. We could hear Roger's mellow voice—and how much he seemed to enjoy it! I could hardly sing for the lump in my throat.

"Oh, that was good! Can we sing another one?" he asked.

"Blessed Assurance" followed. My heart was overwhelmed with the beauty and harmony of family giving heart expression in song! Unknown to me, Marvin had turned on the tape recorder and taped this special time. As the dishes were passed, I noticed that Roger was growing very tired.

He ate a few bites, then said, "Mom, you're going to have to help me out of these clothes!"

I saw everyone glancing at each other in stunned surprise. Was it worth all this? It took about twenty minutes to undress him and pull on his sweats and blankets so he could get warm. In the meantime, the rest of the family finished the meal designed to please Roger.

His eyes followed me around the room. "Thanks, Mom. Everything was so nice and good," he said. It was worth it after all. We took pictures so we wouldn't forget this special evening.

The nighttime hours are long when sleep eludes you, so early morning found him inching his way to the den to a recliner for a change of position, always carrying his afghan with him. Since Marvin is an early riser, it was a good time for father-son chats.

He was pathetically eager to see classmates, teachers, neighbors, and friends, and he requested that we announce an open house for Sunday. Would people feel free to come, knowing of his illness? I didn't want to disappoint him, but I was sure some would fear even casual contact. Yet it would be good for him to have the joy of renewing old friendships. He planned to call and personally invite people. I was reluctant because I feared the rejection. He would not understand this, nor the Midwest mind-set concerning AIDS and gays. He called a good friend as far away as Kansas City. He had not contacted some friends in the past 10 years or so, but now he was eager to see them. I was glad for his interest in friends he had known before he moved to San Francisco.

Friends from our church offered to bring cookies for the open house, while others brought flowers an balloons that added to the festive spirit. Forty people came and offered love and well-wishes. He thoroughly enjoyed it and immediately announced his wish for another such day. I was beginning to be weary and tired from the demands that were required.

Between 35 and 40 persons showed up the second

time to express concern and renew friendship. The sheer joy and excitement that he radiated was well worth the bother.

To confirm his belief that he was being healed he insisted on a repeat of his T-cell ratio, to measure his immune response and defense against viruses. Not only did I think it futile, but wondered if our local hospital lab was prepared to do it. Upon his insistence I called our doctor, who agreed to make arrangements with our laboratory to run the test. Some days later we received the report. It showed no improvement. The T-cell ratio was still very low. He looked at me with sad eyes, not offering any comment, then turned away from me; conversation immediately shifted to another subject.

It was obvious that he was enjoying his days at home. The sunny days in late February were unseasonably warm. He often lay on the porch swing on the patio, basking in the warm sunshine. He was feeling so much better with all the changes that he wanted Dad to bring his typewriter home from the office to see whether he could write his friends in San Francisco. For days he punched keys and completed a letter which Dad copied and which he sent to about 40 people! I helped by addressing the envelopes. In it he somewhat fantasized his ambitions on the premise that he was being healed.

Quoting from his letter:

> As usual, the weather here is predictably unpredictable. Two days ago it was 75 degrees and I was sunbathing on the patio. Today it is 20 degrees and snowing, and they are predicting a blizzard. It is exciting for me, as it has been many years since I have had a direct experience with snow.

> Being with my family has been better than ever. Their way of life is so different, but the bonding of the

extended family is so strong, open, nurturing, and affectionate with each other in a way I never experienced before. I could almost conceive living here some day. *Almost!* It is just such a different way of life. They never lock their doors except at night or when they leave for extended periods of time.

I use this beautiful cane from Russia which some friends of my parents brought for them for a souvenir. I'm convinced it will only be a short time until I will be able to get rid of all canes. "Praise the Lord," as they are saying in these parts.

Roger wished my younger sister, Pearl, from Indiana could come for a visit while he was home. They had been so good to him during his days at Goshen College in Goshen, Indiana. She agreed to come and spend some time with us. But I was beginning to feel bogged down with responsibilities. He couldn't care for himself at all, and demanded much treatment and care. It was so out of character for him to expect anything from anyone for himself, for he'd always been on the giving end. His appetite was very poor and he ate little but thought of many foods he would enjoy. I frantically tried to please and my energy level dropped day by day. His attention span was growing very short and he recognized his inability to think clearly, to remember, or to concentrate.

"My mind just races," he complained.

My sister Joan and friend from Colorado Springs came to spend a long weekend. Roger enjoyed their visit so much. His wish was that we sing together. Music was always a real part of him as it was with my family.

After supper, we gathered around the piano and the old hymnal. With Pearl at the piano we sang four-part harmony page after page. Roger requested that we record it to preserve our time together. Because his voice was so weak, he asked for a microphone so that his part could be heard.

"How Great Thou Art," "Amazing Grace," "Trust and Obey"—we sang for an hour and a half. The memory of that evening will always remain dear to me!

17

Our Times Are in God's Hands

Roger had been home three weeks. We enjoyed the fickle Kansas weather, from sunbathing to snow flurries. Each day brought some surprise or joy. People here are so different, so free, he maintained. It was during the second week that he began to make plans for the future, providing he was healed. He must practice his typing skills, he decided. Perhaps he could get a part-time typing job. I noticed how his hands trembled and wondered how he could imagine himself at the typewriter. He had tried to play the piano but couldn't manipulate his fingers, and had to leave the piano bench in great disappointment. It was difficult for him to sort out reality from fantasy.

One day in the course of our conversation, he learned of a number of sales that were being held downtown. To our surprise he determined to go shopping. How could he—and for what? At first we ignored his request, then realized he was serious. Marvin was reluctant to take him and suggested that Roger should dress up in appropriate clothes for a shopping trip. But, unlike his usual self, he insisted on going as he was, in sweats. Marvin couldn't halt his spending spree and tried to deter him.

Roger jutted his chin out stubbornly. "I know I don't need it, but I want it!"

His reasoning was totally out of character. Yet how can one help when the infected brain cannot give a suitable response? He seemed to be walking better and tolerated more activity. It just didn't make any sense. Again, the nature of AIDS is unpredictable.

He came home from town with two blazers, two pairs of slacks, two pairs of shoes, two shirts, ties, suspenders (red ones at that), a gold ring with a bloodstone, earrings for Mom and Aunt Pearl, and gifts for the girls. The glee in his eyes was that of a delighted child. He apparently used his bankcard. He luckily had sufficient funds to cover the cost, but he would never be able to use any of the items he had bought. It seemed such a waste, but it gave him sheer pleasure to engage in such activity as he had before his illness. The most difficult was in not knowing how to deal with this new set of complications.

One morning during bath time, Roger became very paranoid about continuing on the medication, Acyclovir, a drug given for treatment of herpes, and grew determined to discontinue it. He was experiencing difficulties in vision and was scared of going blind. I encouraged him to continue as prescribed or else he might erupt with another active episode of disease. Finally he agreed to take it once a day, instead of three times daily.

For two days he was in control, then acute symptoms cropped up. Gastrointestinal problems developed, and he remembered the old pattern of previous disorders. His constant fever was more elevated. He ate very little, and I grew anxious about managing his medications. Our doctor did well with the medical history that was available to him.

Friends and relatives provided encouragement and support, but in spite of it all I was beginning to feel very weary . . . physically exhausted . . . tired from daily laundering . . . planning and preparing meals for added guests . . . incessant activity . . . daily visitors . . . being on top of everything—all without finding a quiet time to replenish my spirit. For all this, I felt guilty.

I found comfort in the words of the hymn writer, Henry W. Baker: "Art thou weary, art thou languid." I certainly qualified. I came to Jesus, following his wound prints, and found rest and blessing.

Sometimes I worried about Roger's readiness to die. His racing mind would toy with the question of the certainty of his eternal destination. Was my faith wavering? At times he was not rational at all in his reasoning. I knew he couldn't help it. The Lord promises to give us *himself.* That is all I need!

I began to sense a real restlessness in Roger. He was receiving many phone calls from San Francisco, and he was missing his friends.

One morning he turned to me. "You are very tired and it's time for me to go back home. Do you think you could get a return date for my ticket?"

I felt so guilty again. Could he detect my weariness? I was not wearing my mask very well. As much as I hated to see him leave, it almost seemed like a welcome reprieve. I felt so helpless in knowing how to deal with the problems. How would we make sure that hospice could pick him up again when he got back?

"I don't need hospice anymore," he mumbled when I voiced my concern.

I was aghast! It was obvious that he understood neither his condition nor his real needs. I knew we were in real trouble. How much he would need the support network as soon as he arrived back home!

Marvin checked with the travel agency and reserved a seat for his return in two weeks. We notified hospice of his plans to return and his need for continued care.

His racing thoughts continued, and he requested a professional photographer to take family portraits. It would be our last chance for a family picture, he said. I thought it was a wonderful idea, but at this late date I wondered who would be available.

"Surely you can find someone," he insisted. To my surprise, we were able to get an appointment for the following day.

Roger dressed in his new blazer, slacks, and shoes for what was to be his last dress-up occasion. It was a difficult and lengthy ordeal; a rest period was essential between each pose. We marveled at the results as we later viewed the proofs. The childlike eyes spoke of his illness, but his smile was genuine. We will treasure these portraits forever.

Packing his bags for his return trip became quite an ordeal, with all the extra clothes and shoes. He had also requested that I make him a new red tablecloth for his dining table and matching padded chair backs and seats for his four chairs.

This was all to fit into his suitcase and carry on bag. Medications and treatment paraphernalia nearly filled the carry on case.

My heart ached as I thought of the trauma of his traveling alone, changing planes, waiting in airports, and depending on attendants or whoever was available to assist him. There were too many "what ifs" I could think of. Marvin debated on traveling back with him, but Roger thought the added expense was foolish when he could manage on his own. We made a number of phone calls to California, lining up people to give care and making sure someone was available to pick him up at the airport.

I found my promise in Psalm 37:5 "Commit your way to the Lord; trust in him and he will do this."

I remember the joy and anticipation of his coming. Now I felt heavy with sorrow as he prepared to leave. I was uneasy about his ability to manage this flight. My mother's intuition was later confirmed.

Emotions were high as we said good-bye and watched the attendant push his wheelchair down the ramp. Never again would he return to us.

As the gate was closed a stewardess came to us and asked, "Could you tell us what his illness is so we can better assist him?"

"He had AIDS," Marvin said simply.

She looked stunned and the color drained from her face as she fell back against the wall, which supported her. Without another word she turned, walked down the ramp, and hurried into the plane.

18

Missing Person

We had carefully related the date, arrival time, and flight number to a friend who was to meet him at the airport, and gave instructions to notify us of his safe arrival. The designation time came and went—and stretched into hours. After several frantic phone calls we learned that he was not on the expected plane. Later flights failed to bring him.

Anxious thoughts rushed through our minds. Where was he? What had happened? Passenger agents knew nothing of his whereabouts. I suspected he might have called his Denver friend and met her in the airport on his trip home. I knew only her given name, no address or telephone number.

We were finally able to contact a friend in California who also knew her during college days. After a series of calls, we learned that Roger had missed his plane and lost his ticket. He called his Denver friend, who graciously came and provided him food and shelter for another day.

It was with some fear and trepidation that the friend and her family had accommodated this person who seemed like a stranger. He no longer looked like the Roger they once knew. He was obviously ill. His performance was out of character and his mind was not functioning properly. Were they safe with him? they wondered. AIDS is a fearful disease. How much precaution was needed? Yet out of love and pity they ministered to him and got him on a plane the following day. His bankcard was used a lot those days!

I was able to talk to this friend the following day and she confirmed the rather frightening events. She was cautious in relating his behavior to protect me from embarrassment. I acknowledged her kindness and prayed that God would reward her.

Finally word came that he had arrived home, exhausted but safe. His baggage was on schedule too. A hundred questions pummeled through my mind. How will his care-givers manage this change of behavior? What if there was a break in his support network? Should we have allowed him to return home?

We received reports that he appeared restless. He was aware that he could not control his train of thought. The frustration of trying to maintain his rationality made him very tired. I wearily threw myself at the Lord's feet once more: How often I asked the question: has he not suffered enough? Have I not acted on the belief that you are able to bring peace to those who seek it, Lord? Is there yet some sin in my life that hinders my prayers from being answered? I long for more of yourself. Empty me of anything that might hinder you from living in me. Cleanse me of anything not pleasing to you. Glorify yourself in whatever way you can, using these fragile earthen pots. I will give you the praise and glory. You are a great and mighty God!

Would I ever go to peaceful sleep without a heavy burden? I was always calling on the Lord, it seemed. Truly he was my shelter, my source of strength, my rock of safety!

19

A Call for Help

It was 8:00 p.m. Marvin had an after-supper appointment and would not be home until approximately nine o'clock. Every ring of the telephone seemed fraught with apprehension. When the phone rang, it was Peggy, the hospice coordinator.

"This is an emergency, Helen. I am here at Roger's and I am taking him to San Francisco General Hospital's psychiatric ward and put him on a 72-hour hold until you can get here and decide what you want to do. It's not safe to leave him here any longer. His mind is running like crazy and he needs immediate intervention. Is it possible for you to come right away?"

Her words stunned me. We knew he was confused, but not as much as she seemed to indicate.

"Yes, of course, we'll come as soon as we can," I gulped. "Marvin's not at home. The travel agency and banks are closed, and I'm sure we can't leave before morning. We'll try to get in by the noon flight." My voice shook.

"I'll call back as soon as I can get him admitted and will give you further details." Peggy sounded urgent.

With my face cupped in my hands, I could only sob and plead for wisdom and direction from the Lord.

Quickly I dialed Sheryl's number so they could surround us with prayer. Sheryl's immediate response was that perhaps she should go along, give support, and assist with details. What a comfort she was! Earlier than I expected, Marvin came home. Why hadn't I asked for more details? he asked.

"There wasn't time. She's calling back as soon as she can to tell us more. I sensed that she didn't want to discuss this within Roger's hearing," I told him.

Our local travel agent deserves a medal for all the services she gave us in those months! Marvin called her at home. She went down to the office and issued us tickets at 10:00 p.m. The beautiful people in this town need recognition.

I was becoming proficient at packing bags on a moment's notice. The same few outfits seemed to find their way automatically into the well-worn suitcase. It was always a challenge to keep the laundry done.

We waited for what seemed like an eternity for that return call. Our minds played all kinds of tricks with more questions than solutions. Why did we allow him to return? We couldn't take him home with us now. If hospice couldn't care for him, what alternatives were there? It was almost too much for me to think about. As a nurse I knew he couldn't be hospitalized unless his condition was acute. If only his mind had been spared from the fatal virus. The suffering of his body should have been enough. It was all so unlike him that I could hardly think logically.

Sheryl had decided to go with us. The bags were ready, the tickets in hand, and arrangements made for Leo to take us to the airport. Finally, at 11:30 p.m. the call came. Peggy had admitted him to the psychiatric ward for evaluation and treatment if that was indicated. Insurance would probably pay for 72 hours unless treatment was prescribed, she added.

Then she told us what had happened the past few days. The story went on and on. It was incredible!

"He called a cab to take him shopping," Peggy said. "He bought a big sofa hide-a-bed, a piano, rugs, linens, lamps, and numerous households items. The furniture had been delivered and his apartment barely had walking room left. He tossed some of his furniture down the stairs to the lower level. He had burned candles down to the end, some wooden holders even being charred. He left pots and pans on the stove with the burners turned on, and scorched them. . . ."

I couldn't take in any more information. Where were all the care-givers? I demanded.

Peggy drew a quick breath. "Roger dismissed them because he didn't need them anymore, he said!"

I gasped. He was so ill! How could he have possibly done these things? He couldn't even bathe or dress himself! How could he shop when he could barely totter with assistance? It was all so out of character for him to spend so much money on himself; consideration for others always came first. I shook my head, bewildered. How deadly this awful virus had become!

Peggy's concern was for Roger. She had come to love him too, as had so many who had cared for him. "He is a very special person," was a comment we heard all the time. We were thankful for Peggy and all the other friends.

We were asked to come to the hospice office immediately upon our arrival in San Francisco, at about 1:00 p.m. the next day.

Sleep didn't come easy that night. I tried to recall our conversations with Roger concerning many things. I remembered asking him what he would do when he could no longer live at home. With reluctance he said he would probably have to go to a Shanti home if they had room. I had never heard of such a place and asked more about it. He didn't really know much, he said. He only knew that it was a place to go for those who were ill and homeless for various reasons.

"Some landlords, upon learning that his renter has AIDS, will just throw him out on the street and he has no place to go," he told me. It sounded quite callous to me. I hoped that Roger would always have a safe place to stay.

Early morning we were again on the way to the Wichita airport. It was beginning to feel like familiar turf. We tried to encourage each other. I felt that I was the most needy person in the world. Yet we could trust God to be faithful.

We arrived at Oakland airport on schedule, picked up our rental car, and headed for the San Francisco AIDS hospice office. By now they knew us at the motel and didn't require our bankcard number for holding a room when we phoned in our reservation. The social worker and nurse were waiting for us. After briefing us on events, we were given opportunity to express our wishes concerning Roger's future. What kind of alternatives were there? we asked.

They suggested we apply immediately for admittance to a Shanti residence for neurologically impaired patients. They warned us that there might be a long waiting list. He would need a place where 24-hour care was provided. They also suggested it was likely that he would not be able to stay more than a few days in the hospital, unless they found some acute need for treatment. We would have to plan what to do with him upon his release.

"You may have to stay and care for him yourself," they said.

How could we possibly do this? They said that he could never be cared for in his home anymore. If hospice could not manage that, it was unlikely that we could.

What a blessing to have Sheryl with us! She helped us to be realistic but sensitive and we cautiously planned one step at a time.

Every breath was a prayer as we fought the heavy traffic to the Pride House (Shanti) office in downtown San Francisco. Even the simple act of finding a parking space seemed to require special petition! I'm sure the Lord knew our dilemma and showed us one less than a block away. Office personnel were anticipating our visit. They were warm and cordial, brought us coffee, and offered us comfortable chairs. There was a wealth of reading materials on AIDS, Shanti, support services, and grieving. We felt very much at ease as we waited our turn. It was preparation for us.

After being pleasantly greeted in the coordinator's office, we gave a history of our son's journey with AIDS and his need for admittance. They asked for much detail and data to complete the stacks of paperwork. We were told that there was nothing available now; there was a waiting list, and patients had to die for vacancies to appear.

As we were completing our admission details, Mr. Lister, the director, appeared and asked whether we were the Hostetlers. He wanted to meet us. He was a soft-spoken, gracious gentleman. He said he had been in touch with Dr. Bair from San Francisco General, who requested that space and immediate care be provided for Roger. He said he wanted to assure us that they would be able to admit him in about three weeks!

I was so moved that I couldn't speak. Talk about a great God! How could we thank these people enough? Miracles indeed do happen. Feebly and with emotion, we tried to offer our thankfulness.

We completed admitting details and headed for San Francisco General Hospital. How would we find Roger?

20

The Chill of Chains

We were being given directions to San Francisco General Hospital. Our rental car took us on a roller-coaster ride through a maze of traffic racing to who knew where. It took all three of us, watching for landmarks, lights, and street signs, to keep from a collision. I always marveled how we were able to end up at our destination. Our guardian angels were working overtime.

When we reached the hospital, we were surrounded by sirens, ambulances, and police officers. We pushed our way toward the hospital entrance. For a moment I thought I was dreaming . . . then I wished I were. After weaving through a maze of people, some crying, some cursing, some hemorrhaging, some vomiting, others demonstrating fitful behavior . . ., we stepped into the elevator with directions to the psychiatric ward. I felt as though we had already passed through it.

We passed through a large garden area into a huge foyer and found ourselves in front of a large bolted door. There was no handle on the door and no one to give us further directions.

As I looked around, chills enveloped my body. I didn't know whether to cry, scream, or run. Through the barred windows we saw a similar door with a very small room in between. After standing there for a few minutes, puzzled, we noticed a panel which appeared like a speaker with a button below it. Marvin decided it was the communicator, and bravely pushed the button.

Soon a male voice said, "What's your name?"

"Marvin Hostetler."

"Step in and register."

With that we heard a loud buzzing sound. Marvin pushed the door that opened and then shut behind us, and we found ourselves locked in the small room.

Through the barred window we saw people pacing back and forth, some staring into space. One large woman waved her arms and let out a bloodcurdling scream. We heard considerable commotion in the background.

No words can express the emotion I experienced. Roger doesn't belong in a place like this! He is so ill. These people are mentally sick, but Roger is ill in his physical body. My heart pounded so loud that I could hear it. My arms were covered with goose bumps, and I shook. I breathed a prayer: Please God, let me feel your presence. Assure me of your safekeeping. We need your wisdom, your love. I need your comfort right now. . . .

I could feel a warm glow enveloping my body. Truly the Lord was even in this place! He brought to my mind commissioning words from Isaiah 61:1-3:

> The spirit of the Lord God is upon me, because the Lord has anointed me to bring good tidings to the afflicted; He has sent me to bind up the brokenhearted, to proclaim liberty to the captives . . . to comfort all who mourn . . . to give a garland instead of ashes . . . gladness instead of mourning . . . praise instead of a faint heart. (RSV)

An amazing calmness came over me. Because of God, we truly had love and comfort to give.

My thoughts were interrupted by the jangle of keys in the door and a man stood before us.

"Whom do you wish to see?" he asked.

"Roger Hostetler."

"Please sign the register and come with me."

He told us that two hours a day were allowed for immediate family to visit, but since Roger was a "different" patient we could probably spend as much time as we wished.

He led the way down a long hall to a barred room with a single bed and bedside table. There were no curtains or drapes, no pictures or chairs, just a bed with not enough covers. Our eyes met Roger's, and with eyes blurred, our arms were around each other. Water dripped from the ceiling. He had asked us to place his towel to soften the drips that were annoying him. In tears he told us the nightmare of being in this place.

"I don't think I belong here. I know my mind isn't working right, but I'm not really crazy!" he muttered.

My heart went out to him. In the background we could hear screaming, cursing, and filthy language. He said he was *expected to do his own laundry* even though he was not able to do it. He asked us to bring him more clothes. Then his brow furrowed.

"I can't understand Peggy. Why did she send me here?" he cried.

We tried to explain the concern that others had for his safety, and that they were admitting him for tests to determine the possibility of a chemical imbalance that might be treatable. He was here for diagnosis and therapy, we emphasized. We told him that he was here because they cared about him. (I tried to make myself believe it!)

We were allowed to assist him into the day room to a sofa. The environment was less depressing and away from the distracting drips. The activity here was at times amusing, sometimes sad and distracting, and other times a bit frightening. Patients took us to be everything from notables to suspicious derelicts. We were never sure whether we should talk to them or remain quiet and aloof. I was sure no normal person could be in that ward for 24 hours and maintain his sanity!

Roger requested that we do our best to get him out of the place. Why couldn't he be admitted to a regular hospital ward? he asked. One floor was devoted to the care of AIDS patients. The questions seemed logical. We assured him we had an appointment with the doctors the next morning and would do our best. At the Shanti office it was suggested that the doctors should prepare the patient to accept entrance into the Shanti homes. It should be a voluntary admittance on the part of the patient. It was hard to deal with the facts. Roger would know that this transfer would mean giving up his home—and that this was a place to go to await death. How much more could we take? I couldn't bear that thought. We noticed his attention span was short. The conversation shifted from one subject to another in rapid succession. It was hard to develop a train of thought. At the same time he was oriented, alert, and very much aware what was going on.

We were allowed to bring in meals and eat with him, for who could eat alone in this environment? A friendly gentleman shuffled through the ward, offering us oranges or apples. He picked up trash, arranged chairs, and we couldn't figure out whether he was an attendant or a patient! The second day our suspicions were confirmed that he was a patient.

We decided to eat with Roger as often as reasonable. Wes, a faithful hospice volunteer, came regularly to see him, offer his love and care, and eat with us. His presence was heartwarming. He was helping to bear our burdens. Many other friends were given visiting privileges because Roger was a "special" patient. He had a quality that endeared himself to all, including patients on that ward.

At the motel we awoke early the next morning to the roar of traffic far below us on Highway 101, but the beauty of the sunrise was breathtaking. The eastern sky was aflame in shades of brilliant reds and golds. We could see the reflection in the bay directly below us. Marvin opened the drapes wide for us to catch the beauty. Our visiting hours were scheduled for afternoons so we would make the most of the mornings.

On the way to Roger's house we discovered a McDonalds which became our routine breakfast stop for a bran muffin and coffee. Marvin found that a ham and cheese McMuffin was suitable for his diabetic diet. It was clearly the cheapest place to eat.

When we pulled up in front of Roger's house we were sad. Reluctantly we got out of the car. Marvin unlocked the outer gate and approached the door. There was no reason to ring the doorbell with our code. No one would be there to answer. Inside the foyer we found a casserole dish with a note:

> 4/8/86—Hostetlers:
>   Here's a sort of made-up casserole—rice, chicken, broccoli, etc. It just needs to be heated. Also, the paper re SSI and Disability from Pac Bell was with some mail Roger gave me last week.
>
> Doug

The lump in my throat was so big that I couldn't swallow.

"Bless his heart," Sheryl said.

As if he hadn't already done enough! But how very thoughtful. It would be all we would need for the day.

Doug was that special person who had the burden of taking care of Roger's business, paying his bills, and trying to keep the debits and credits in balance. Sheryl called him an oasis in the desert. We shared his time, his love, and his prayers. Later in the week, he invited us along with other friends to a lovely dinner in the apartment he shared with John. The formal table was beautifully set with lace and flowers. Classical music formed the background for a very relaxed, quiet, and beautiful evening. The tasty three-course dinner was served with grace. We will never forget this act of love. It provided a much-needed diversion from our difficult task.

As we entered Roger's house and started toward the living room, we couldn't believe our eyes. Everything was in disorder. We found it just as Peggy had said. Where do we begin to clean up, we wondered?

Marvin surveyed the situation and began making suggestions. We decided to go through everything carefully. We had the list of things that he wanted to give to friends and family. Everything would be carefully boxed and labeled. We also had a list of personal things that were allowed in the Shanti residence. We wanted him to have as much there as possible to make it feel like home. What should we do with his many plants?

Beginning with the sun-room, we removed everything and disposed of the fiber carpet. We scrubbed and waxed the vinyl that was under it, then stacked the sorted boxes there. Marvin had a way of running into the right people at the right time. He noticed the Salvation Army truck several blocks down the street. The drivers were having a coffee break, and he made arrangements for them to pick up the bed, two mattresses, pillows, and old bedding.

We tried to determine what was special to Roger and take it to his hospital room. It turned out later that we had made some good choices.

It was obvious that the house had not been thoroughly cleaned in a long time. The collections of a lifetime, even at 35 years, are numerous. There were a number of undesignated items such as pots, pans, and a whole library of records and books.

How thankful we were for Doug's casserole. At noon we stuck it in the microwave for a few minutes and lunch was ready.

For the next three days we cleaned and packed, interspersed with visits to the hospital. Roger was aware of what we were doing, and it was difficult for him. He knew what he had and where it was located. He asked us to detail it all for him, which we did. I tried to put myself in his place, but it was too painful. How could we be so cruel as to make plans to vacate his apartment and dispose of all his belongings? We assured him we would not do it until he made the move to the Shanti residence. I could never have gone through this experience without Sheryl's help.

Each time we returned to the hospital, Roger asked for a report. Things we had considered worthless to anyone were crammed into large garbage bags. On this particular day, he asked us to bring the quilt I had made for him which he had been using as a throw over his one occasional chair in the bedroom. Sheryl and I looked at each other and gulped. The top was pieced with brightly colored scraps. It was badly soiled, and I didn't think it would stand washing, so we had tossed it into a garbage bag along with discarded medications and ointments, spoiled food, broken candles, and numerous other disposables.

"I . . . threw it away," I confessed.

"But it was my most prized cover!" he wailed. I couldn't believe his anguish at losing that cover.

Dad tried to explain to no avail. We decided we'd try to retrieve it. Marvin didn't want to dig it out, but I felt obligated at least to search for it. If we found it, we could always dispose of it later.

Sure enough, we found it but it was filthier than ever, from other things that had been piled on top of it. We placed it in a separate bag and stashed it in his closet. When we told him we had found it, he was like a child that had recovered a broken, treasured toy. I began to feel his sorrow at losing everything, family, friends, and possessions.

The following day we met with the team of doctors for his evaluation. Rosemary, who had agreed to be his durable power of attorney for health care, also met with us. With apprehension we walked into that conference room. The medical team demonstrated dignity and concern as they related their findings and suggested supportive care rather than active therapy. The AIDS virus had done neurological damage and there was no known treatment to reverse this, they told us. They anticipated progression of the disease and deterioration of all systems. He would never be able to care for himself and he would need consistent 24-hour care. The only solution they knew was admittance to a Shanti residence with hospice care. They had been in touch with the Shanti director, who had advised them of the probability of admitting Roger within three weeks. The hospital would keep him until then.

This report was not unexpected but nevertheless it made us sad. Roger agreed to the proposal. But wait three more weeks? His face fell. We assured him of daily phone calls and the possibility of a transfer sooner.

21

Courage in Times of Testing

A week had come and gone. Plans had been finalized for Roger's continued care and we were able to spend most of the days with him. To him, it seemed the time was never long enough. To feel needed, wanted, and loved, warms any heart. For us it was especially precious because it came from a dear son whose giving would soon be gone forever. We had so much love to give. Plans to dispose of property and give up his apartment concerned us and were hard for Roger to deal with. Now with newly purchased furnishings how could we make plans that would not break Roger's heart? He seemed less able to deal with death than previously.

One day I asked him what was different and what had changed since the night of his celebration party, when he had chosen to share with his friends the peace he had and his wish to go to heaven.

He looked at me with deep searching eyes and said, "I don't know."

I knew that due to neurological impairment, his level of comprehension was far from normal, and he wasn't accountable for what he couldn't handle. He continued to talk about his ambitions and plans to do things—always to help someone. He shared his dreams of wanting to be a physician's assistant so he could help people with AIDS. Or he wanted to brush up his typing skills and help in the office—not on the payroll, but just as a volunteer until he could get better!

His nights were long and sleepless. He reported on the restless activities of other patients on the ward at night.

Among his papers I found a letter written to a friend while he was confined to the ward. It was very difficult to interpret. He wanted me to type it and mail it. I lacked a typewriter and time, forgot the address, and could never fulfill his wish. The letter follows:

Dear Patty:

So nice to hear from you again. Just wanted you to know that I am locked up in the city mental ward. It is a horrible place and very depressing for me. Over the past few months my mind has been deteriorating rapidly. I'm here for neurological profile, hoping that my absent-mindedness is due to a chemical imbalance that can be cured with a drug.

It's hard for me to have given up *all* my freedom. I get an allowance each week from my power of attorney, and that's all I can spend. It's okay. Anything is okay. My parents are here again, but I can only have visitors two hours a day, so I hardly see them.

Pray that I survive the ordeal and share this with your family and friends. My telephone number is 415-555-9307 if you ever feel like calling. I'll probably be in the hospital for a long time.

Much love,
Roger

I thought of how much he suffered silently. He was never free of physical pain. He constantly suffered a severe headache and elevated temperature. Because of the peripheral neuropathy just touching his arms or body caused pain. Sometimes I forgot this as I hugged him and was reminded as I heard him groan. Gastrointestinal problems were always present and psoriasis a constant discomfort.

More than the physical pain was the emotional agony. We were not aware of the intense pain he had suffered the past few years—the need always to guard relationships lest there be more rejection. Oh, how I wish he could have felt free to share his deep, troubled emotions, without feeling we were judging him. If only we had known how to be more helpful. It was not unlike the inner hurt he often suffered before his illness.

The following is a journal entry dated September 9, 1985, soon after his return from Bali:

> It was so beautiful and wonderful, an experience of love and acceptance not unlike Bali. Also Shell Beach was so peaceful and beautiful that it was always somehow nurturing just to be there. In my desire to stay there, I realized that I was just procrastinating getting on with my life here. I have such a strong will to attain my goal that something is bound to work out.

> I'm feeling frustrated at even relating to my friends here. Everyone seems so caught up in whatever it is we get caught up in. I just want to learn more about that carefree and effortless existence which enables the Balinese friends to *give* so much. I don't think of any reason why I should have anything less than this sort of experience in my life.

> It's already difficult for me to remember with any clarity how it felt to really love myself as I recall my experience in Bali. I remember the impact, but the actual experience is fading.

> I still feel rather frail and vulnerable. It's disgusting to have to start building back the walls that I let down completely over there. To begin to have to shut people out in order to protect myself. It was so liberating to operate without them. . . .

Praise God, he had now experienced acceptance from his parents and was able to share his feelings, but with such suffering. We now needed to provide for him a place of complete freedom and peace for which he so much longed. His present racing mind gave him no rest.

I was thankful for the kind way the team of doctors had approached Roger with their suggested care plan, which included residency in a Shanti home. They assured him that they had his best interest at heart. Their credibility impressed Roger, and he responded favorably, knowing, of course, that there were no other options. The hospice volunteers whom he had learned to love and trust would be able to continue with his care.

On the day before our return flight, we were visiting Roger in the day room in the morning. Dr. Bair came over and asked to speak with us. What news was waiting for us now?

With a troubled look on her face, she said, "A complication has come up. We have notice that Roger will not be able to stay here any longer. His health insurance will not pay for any additional days, and we know that it's impossible for you or any private party to pay for this kind of hospitalization. He didn't qualify for continuance because he was not being treated for an acute infectious process, and the testing and diagnosis has been completed. How long will you be staying?"

"We have a return ticket and reservation for early in the morning," Marvin said.

"Can you be back here at 3:30 this afternoon? We'll see what we can do until then," the doctor added.

I could not believe my ears! I knew God wouldn't let us down now. There had to be a way. We needed to keep our anxieties from Roger. It was necessary for us to leave to collect our thoughts and pray.

In the meantime, the hospice office was trying to reach us. We discovered they had been given the same notice we were given. It was Friday. The office would be closed for the weekend, and we were to call them back before five o'clock. We could not leave without definite plans for Roger's care. What should we do?

Marvin got on the phone to family and friends at home, asking for special prayer for guidance and decision-making. Prayer chains were asked to pray in our behalf. I had to believe God would provide a solution. I was reminded of the passage in 1 Corinthians 10:13: "God is faithful, and he will not let you be tempted beyond your strength" (RSV).

I will not give in to panic and despair. I will believe for a solution, I decided.

Back at the hospital, we went directly to the conference room to wait for the doctors.

After greetings, Dr. Bair spoke? "Roger can stay here until he can be transferred to the Shanti residence. We have resubmitted a verification of need. If that does not qualify him, we have found a way that city funding will provide for his extended stay."

Again we were overwhelmed! I couldn't speak. My eyes were full of tears.

"Oh, thank you. Thank you, Lord! We can never tell you how grateful we are." It was all I could say.

I glanced at my watch, hunted a telephone, and reported to the hospice office before closing time. Lorna, the social worker, was waiting for our call. I told her the news as it was given to us. There was a long silence at the other end of the phone line.

"Are you there?" I asked.

Another pause. "Yes . . . but . . . I have never heard of such a thing!"

"It's from our great God," I cried. "I believe it's a miracle. It's the Lord's doing and we are *so* grateful."

"Well, I am too . . ." was all she could say. Then she went on. "Now that we know this, I can tell you that it will not be longer than three weeks, maybe not even two. The person that Roger will replace is very near death. I don't see how he can last more than a week. I am so glad you were able to work it out for your son. It will be a good place for him."

She gave me the address so we could drive by if we wished. We told her that we would be back in two weeks to clean out his apartment and dispose of his belongings to designated persons.

This last time we could visit Roger in peace. We didn't tell him of our hectic but otherwise marvelous, eventful day!

He was happy for the news that we would be returning soon and he could count the days. He begged us to try to get him out of the hospital. We assured him of daily phone calls and that the time would pass quickly. Perhaps he could be an inspiration to someone there, I suggested. The day that he could be released would not come soon enough, we were sure.

The evening passed quickly. We had brought dinner to eat with him, but none of us were very hungry.

Parting time seemed easier than usual. We promised to be back soon. For Sheryl it was more difficult, since it would probably be the last time she would see him.

Good-bye forever had been said before, but this time it seemed different. Marvin and I started for the exit and waited. I could see Sheryl tenderly holding him close. As she left him, his sad eyes followed her. When we turned toward the door, he lifted his thin hand and waved farewell.

The test came as we left through the double-barred, locked doors. I turned to get a last glimpse and met his sorrowful eyes as he lay on the sofa in the day room wrapped in his many covers. With a wave of the hand we were out of sight.

22

Anxious Waiting

The days that followed were difficult. Roger had access to the pay phone on the ward. He had misplaced his Day-Timer, in which he kept telephone numbers, addresses, and appointments. He couldn't remember familiar and oft-used numbers. In his loneliness, he tried to call numerous friends across the country. Many were collect calls. Finally the staff had to request that calls be limited. This added to his feelings of confinement. We assured him that he could always call us and that we would call every morning at eight o'clock, so he could depend on that.

The calls became more and more frequent, often three and four times a day.

"Can't I please come home? I just need to be where you are," he pleaded through sobs. Can you imagine how these would tear a mother's heart to shreds?

Or, "Could I go to Sheryl or Janene's?"

One day he called Janene. She gave in to his request and said he could come. Then she panicked. Yet how could she let him come? She would so much have liked to honor his wish.

"Couldn't the relatives take turns and relieve you so it wouldn't be so hard on you?" he begged, his voice raw with pleading.

I couldn't bear it. I tried, against my better judgment, to convince Marvin that we could manage some way. For long we had wished to have him home more often and for longer periods of time. Now when he wanted to be with us, couldn't we honor his wish? How tragic. Then we would get calls from his care-givers, reminding us that we could never provide the services he required.

"Couldn't I go to The Cedars of Showalter Villa?" he pleaded knowing that nursing homes took care of bed-fast patients. I couldn't tell them that they wouldn't take him even if they had empty rooms. There is still fear and lack of education in the Midwest concerning the care of AIDS patients.

He couldn't understand that his requests were impossible to consider even though we wanted it to be otherwise. (A couple years later both home health care and hospice were ready to care for AIDS patients in our county. I am proud of the effort that has been put forth to educate and to give aid as well. It was too late for us.)

Even at this point in his illness, he longed for the pleasure of normal family experiences.

One day he spilled out his heart in sobbing, "If only I could have been straight! I would so much have loved to have a family of my own and children to love. Will you forgive me for the heartaches I've caused you?"

How my heart ached for him. His yearning was so genuine. With every phone call the first and last greeting was always, "I love you" or "I love you so much." The conversations were brief. He would tire very easily, but he also fantasized about "having a job" and earning money to pay his bills. He would relate activities on the ward, usually by some disruptive patient. He could not sleep, he claimed.

We had promised to return in two weeks and he was counting the days. He felt that when we got there, all his troubles would be over; we could make anything better. He was concerned about his personal business and getting all the bills paid; he was fearful that things were not properly cared for when he couldn't do them himself.

He finally realized the he could not keep the furniture he had purchased, but making a decision about disposition was very difficult.

Every day he'd beg, "Please hurry and come. Can't you come sooner? Pray for me." Sometimes a call would come in the middle of the night. He didn't realize what time of day or night it was or he would forget that he had just called.

Marvin was busy making plans for bringing home the things he wished us to have. He designed and built a folding carrier for the rental car, to get baggage to the airport. He purchased a foot locker for storage of large articles. We mailed notices to his friends that we would be at his apartment between 2:00 and 4:00 p.m. on Saturday and Sunday so they could pick up their gifts. For the first time we planned in advance to purchase tickets at a reduced fare.

Friends from First Mennonite Church in McPherson were very special. I don't know how we would have survived without them. We received calls of encouragement, assurance of prayer, and appropriate cards to acknowledge their care. They learned we were planning a return trip.

One morning our church treasurer stopped by on his way to work and handed us an envelope. It was a gift from the church, he said, to help with our expenses. We were overwhelmed and choked up. We had never questioned God's provisions, but the perfect timing of this need was mind-boggling. Our funds were exhausted. We always knew it was better to give than to receive. Now we knew what it was like to allow others to help. We were deeply grateful.

There were other times of tenderness when friends came to encourage and give gifts in times of real need. I especially remember the time a dear friend came to our door.

"I know that it was by God's design that I ran into you today uptown and learned of your need to make a trip to California again. God showed me that you needed this. We want you to use it as you see fit," she said as she closed my had over a bill. In a fumbling way I tried to express our thanks, and when I looked at the large bill, I was overcome with their love.

Many times I have asked God to bless and reward them for such sensitivity and faithfulness to God. It is a rich but humbling experience to learn to receive.

The burden of care was always before me. How thankful I am for the Scripture I memorized in my younger years. The familiar words of Jesus came to me in such a comforting way:

> Come to me, all who labor and are heavy laden, and I will give you rest. Take my yoke upon you, and learn from me; for I am gentle and lowly in heart, and you will find rest for your souls. For my yoke is easy, and my burden is light. (Matthew 11:28-30, RSV)

The invitation is so simple—*Come, I will give you rest.* I would ask in faith, believing that the Lord would carry my burden. I was tired in body and broken in spirit, and the weight was breaking me down. I literally raised my hands and gave it all to God. "It's now for you to carry, Lord. Roger belongs to you. It is for you to do with him what you will. I can do nothing." I wept and praised God, and the burden lifted. I felt free! The release was indescribable.

Early one morning we received the call. "Hi, Mom. I love you. Guess what? I'm going to move today."

I had learned not to get too excited about any new information because it usually was a fantasy.

"You are?"

"Yes, Jeff is going to move me to the Shanti home."

"Do you have a release?"

"Yes. Aren't you excited about it?" He must have sensed that my response wasn't too enthusiastic.

"What time are you leaving?" I asked finally.

"In the afternoon after work. Rosemary was going to move me, but it's sooner than they planned, and she has to work. I can't wait!"

The information rolled across my mind and I wondered if it were true. "Call us when you get settled and tell us about it," I suggested.

Another call followed that morning with the same information. Again I acknowledged the good news. Marvin was also on the line and gave him some words of cheer and told him he was delighted. This time I was beginning to believe it.

I was sitting at the dinner table gazing out across the patio into the back lawn and watched a plump robin pluck a worm out of the fresh green grass. It was a bright spring day. The crocuses and daffodils were starring the grass with nuggets of gold, and the air was scented with growing things. There was evidence of new life everywhere. It gave one a feeling of resurrection after a long cold winter. I needed that feeling of newness.

The phone rang, and I continued to sit for a moment. Staring at the phone, I momentarily wished I didn't have to answer it. Finally I lifted the receiver after another ring.

"This is Doug. I just wanted to let you know that Ruth and I moved Roger to the Shanti residence this afternoon."

My heart raced with the good news, and I hated myself for not having shown more excitement to Roger this morning. In a rather humorous fashion Doug related the fun of trying to pack into his compact car, along with three riders, all Roger's collection of clothes, bedding, flowers, and assorted paraphernalia he had accumulated from his friends during his hospital stay. Doug's report was most encouraging. He said the house was beautiful, a typical Victorian home. Roger's room was adequate with nice furniture, but most of all he was impressed with the care-givers. The nurses and attendants gave him unusual attention. He had only good things to say and felt that Roger felt greatly relieved to be there. I was exuberant. I couldn't wait to tell Marvin.

Ruth Buxman, pastor of the First Mennonite Fellowship of San Francisco, had accompanied him. She had come with Doug on several visits prior to his hospital release. Roger had taken a real liking to her and, from then on, she became his spiritual mentor. In the several weeks that followed, he became very dependent on her and she very ably ministered to him. The Lord had chosen her to be the person who would gently guide Roger to peace with God and himself.

23

The Healing Team

Once again it was time to pack our suitcases. We needed more detailed planning and preparation to bring home those treasures Roger had given us. It would probably be our last visit, and we sensed the need of being emotionally prepared.

Friends called to pray with us. Pastor Ed Stucky and his wife, Doris, very faithfully came or called before we left each time. Their support meant so much to us.

We had been told that Roger's condition was deteriorating rapidly. Keepsakes needed to be wrapped cautiously to prevent breakage or damage. Marvin decided that we would carry five suitcases and foot locker in our old '69 van and store it at the Wichita airport until our return a week later. Thus we wouldn't need to depend on anyone else for transportation and still have ample room for the extra luggage.

Day was just breaking that Friday as we again left home for another unknown. We had talked of whens, wheres, hows, whys, and what-ifs. It was all in God's hands. He had been so gracious and we recounted how he had provided and blessed.

About 10 miles from the airport I looked up and I saw a brilliant double rainbow! Tears streamed down my cheeks, for I knew without doubt that it was especially for us, since there had been no rain and no hint of the usual reason for rainbows. It was as though God was saying, "Don't worry. I'll look after you." It was a *double promise*. Thank you, Lord.

I checked all our empty suitcases on our tickets and received confirmation of seat assignments while Marvin parked the van in the long-term parking area. After a leisurely cup of coffee we walked to the boarding area and soon we were on our way to Oakland.

As we lifted up above the clouds, I marveled at the power of flying with a load of some 100 passengers plus luggage, freight, and fuel—at 535 miles per hour and 35,000 feet high. Hardly a drop compared to the power of God, I thought. I picked up the emesis bag in the pocket in front of me and began to scribble.

> *May 8, 1986:* "What he hath promised, he is able to perform" (Rom. 4). Another journey, another crisis, another heartache. Will it ever come to a peaceful conclusion? How long, O Lord, will you withhold the peace you have promised to give? How long we have prayed for Roger's salvation! Such yearnings for peace. Such desire for rest— complete rest. Such searching for that which satisfies— completely satisfies. He has read the philosophers, traveled the world, experimented with useless habits. He yearned to belong, to feel secure, to be accepted, to be recognized for who he was. He wanted freedom—to be free from what?
>
> How many nights were full of tears? Are you there, Lord? How long before you answer our prayers! Have I yet some hidden sin, some unfinished task I must do before you hear me? In your *own time*, and in your own way, you *will* do your work and will in Roger.
>
> Lord, I believe. Help thou my unbelief. You have given your word. It is stronger than a blade of steel, a two-edged

sword. How swiftly it pierces the defensive armor of life with love. Let my touch be your touch. Love through me. None of me but *all* of thee.

Thank you for the rainbow this morning. We left the airport in the old faithful van with six suitcases nested in each other plus a trunk. They will become receptacles of our son's treasures. No longer will he be able to enjoy the comforts of home. His request was to share all his belongings with family and friends. Precious mementos of life and love we had shared with one so dear—our only son.

The rainbow was God's sign to us this morning, the sign of his promise to us of unending faithfulness. What an emotional, breathtaking moment when we noticed it! He will never forsake us. He will never leave us comfortless. He will answer our prayers.

We have given Roger over to you, Lord. Complete the work in him. He belongs to you. You have given him to us, and we have given him back to you. Blessed be the name of the Lord!

Make the joy of meeting again a warm, loving, sweet occasion. Send your Spirit before us. Anoint us with your presence. Calm Roger's troubled spirit. I know you can. I know you will. "Whatsoever you ask in faith believing, you shall receive."

A miracle? We ask for one. Allow your Spirit to touch him. Allow him to experience your *complete* forgiveness. Your presence with him will give rest and peace and assurance. Thank you, Lord.

The plane is high above the clouds. Big, billowy, white, fluffy clouds are below us. The sun has edged its curls in gold. "How majestic is your name in all the earth."

I dropped my pen and lay my head back in quiet meditation. I was at peace.

After a two-hour layover in Phoenix we again boarded the plane for our final flight to Oakland. We had made reservations for our rental car. It was within easy access to the deplaning area and in a short time we were on our way to San Francisco and the Bayside Motor Lodge. It had become our home away from home.

Employees at the coffee shop now knew us by name and asked about Roger when we arrived.

We left our luggage and fought traffic to the Shanti residence. Our concern was finding a parking place, but the Lord provided a space within the block. Parking was difficult on the steep hill.

We eagerly approached the entrance door. Marvin rang the bell in his usual code, three short bells. Very soon, the door opened and there stood Roger to greet us! With a joyous yell, he hugged us again and again.

"I'm so glad you came," he repeated, then showed us to his room.

Directly to the right of the entry was a large living room. We walked down a long hall. On either side were bedrooms for residents. At the end of the hall was the nurses' station and kitchen. On the far side of the kitchen, a door led to a small patio area with steps to a large deck on the lower level. There were comfortable lounge chairs for resting and relaxing in the sun.

I was pleasantly surprised at the nicely furnished bedroom. Many bouquets and flower arrangements covered the large, double dresser. Several helium balloons with "Happy Birthday" and "We love you" were tied to plants and flowers. On the coffee table were more bouquets. Roger had had a birthday on May 4, and it was evident that his friends had given him a party. A small sofa added to the comfortable furnishings.

On his coffee table his player was softly sounding out his favorite tape, *Dino—Just Piano.* He immediately began telling us of the events of the past week and of his wishes for his Bali painting and wall hangings. He had done some detailed colored pencil drawings before he became too ill and wanted them tacked on the wall. He also wanted more clothes.

"Make a list," he said, and I drew out my pen and paper. Being the detailed person he was, he wanted to be sure I jotted everything down. He even planned outings with us. I could hardly imagine it!

I had fried two chickens, carefully packed in my carrying case, because I knew how well he relished fried chicken.

"Tomorrow I'd like to go to Stowe Lake in Golden Gate Park, and take a picnic lunch," he said.

I wondered if that was possible, but attendants informed me that I had cooking privileges in the kitchen. Each resident had his own food, which was carefully coded. Each was responsible for his own food supply. Aids or attendants prepared meals and snacks according to the patient's request whenever it was desired.

Lorna, the hospice social worker, had called us before leaving and requested a meeting with all the care-givers as soon as we arrived. This included Shanti and hospice aides and volunteers plus friends and family. She would be there to chair the meeting. The purpose was to shape a care program that all understood and make definite plans for meeting Roger's immediate needs. About ten persons were involved in this meeting.

The first item of concern was his wrestling with not being able to forgive himself. There were so many regrets, so much remorse. How were they going to deal with this?

I too had regrets. Who among us doesn't? I regretted

that I had failed to be sensitive to his and others' needs, that I did not always *respond* in love to those who are unlovable. At times I had acted to please myself, or hadn't shared in the burdens of others. And at times I had not allowed the Holy Spirit to control my life. How often I too had been in need of forgiveness!

The simple yet profound act of confession was what we needed to start the process of being recreated into a new and peaceful life. We were experiencing the difficult sorrow of Roger not being allowed to live out life here and now. Because we are mortal, we could not see the beauty of life beyond death. Oh, my son, how I wish I could take your place! was the cry of my heart.

No one there quite understood the problem. Finally Doug said that Ruth Buxman had been making progress with Roger on this issue. She had spent hours with him, he frequently asked her to come, and she had come every day.

We were told that he frequently wanted to go out to eat, then found he could not sit up from fatigue and begged to lie down. We agreed that no one would take him out for meals.

He also wished for a telephone. It was concluded that a private phone would not be to his best interests, but he was allowed to use the staff phone for short visits. This was to avoid unnecessary and frequent calls plus a large bill.

We were also told we could eat with him there. Eating in his room was inconvenient. Using the staff dining room was also disruptive. Since he wanted so much to go to Stowe Lake just once more, the staff agreed to that. We would pack a lunch and take him. He requested butterscotch pudding, potato salad, and chicken. I found it awkward to cook in an unfamiliar kitchen with limited resources where several others also cooked, but

Roger was pleased with my menu. The butterscotch pudding recipe found its way into the staff cookbook for future use!

As we got into the car, Roger suggested that we stop and pick up Ruth to go with us. Since she lived near the Golden Gate Park it seemed like a good idea. She was happy to join us.

The beauty of the park was breathtaking. Masses of flowers added a riot of color everywhere. The well-groomed shrubs and bushes, with a variety of trees in the background, attracted a host of bright, chittering birds.

We found the perfect spot: an alcove on the lake with a backdrop of flowers and trees. I spread out our blanket; pillows, blankets, and afghans for Roger; and our basket of food. He looked around in appreciation for this earthly paradise. His profound fatigue was already obvious. I tried to get him comfortable, then prepared his plate of food. He immediately began to eat as I arranged the food for the rest of us. Before we had begun to eat, he said he had to leave, that he was too tired. We quickly choked down a few bites and gathered up everything so that we could go. Getting him back into the car was like trying to manipulate a rag doll.

He closed his eyes and paid no attention as we returned to his residence.

But it was worth all the effort to grant him this last wish, even though it was not what he anticipated. He knew now that he would never be able to go out for anything again.

We spent the afternoon with him in his room, just being with him, touching, loving, reminiscing. Over and over he wanted the *Dino Praise II* tape played. the beauty of the hymn tunes was quieting and peaceful for him. The tape had been handled so much that the lettering was faded. It was also a comfort to me. He would hum along with: "Sometimes Allelulia," "Sweet Sweet Spirit," and "Leaning on the Everlasting Arms." What power there was in the message!

We decided to let the staff prepare and serve his evening meal, since we needed to get away for a little while. The strain was telling on us.

When we returned Marvin decided to stay and visit with a number of Roger's friends who were in the living room. I went back to his room. After we exchanged the usual hugs and greetings, he said immediately,

"Mom, I want you to pray."

I looked around the room at several others who were there, and for a moment I felt uneasy. Mark, who was his Shanti counselor and emotional support volunteer, was there; we had grown to appreciate him.

"Would you like for Mark to pray?" I asked hesitantly.

"No, I want you to pray," Roger insisted.

I sat on the edge of the bed, took his hand in mine, closed my eyes, and began talking to my heavenly Father. I don't remember the exact words but I thanked him for life, for allowing us to share this time with Roger, for the gift of salvation, for taking our sins, cares, and burdens; for these care-givers and for the love of friends and family. I asked for relief from pain, for healing, and for forgiveness.

As I looked up through misty eyes, I noticed that others had joined us around his bed. I felt as though a spiritual cloak had been wrapped around us all. It was a warm feeling of love and strength. I wouldn't soon forget it.

As the evening progressed, one by one his friends, who had become *our* friends, left. The three of us were alone. Sometimes we laughed, sometimes we felt sad, and sometimes we were just quiet. But it felt good simply to be close to one another. I would treasure every moment.

At one point a sweet, chocolaty aroma filled the room as an attendant came in and treated us to chocolate cupcakes, freshly baked. It was just one of those wonderful things that these dear ones did to make life a bit more pleasant and share their love with little surprises. The staff displayed a glowing spirit, were very compassionate, enthusiastic, full of energy, as well as uplifting. We learned and grew from observing the care demonstrated by both paid and volunteer workers.

One of the purposes for our coming was to clean out his apartment so it could be redecorated and prepared for rental, but we needed to discuss this with Roger. It was a painful subject which we wished we could avoid. He had already suggested a plan for action. We had agreed to spend the afternoon of the following day at his house, giving personal things to designated people who would be there to pick them up.

When we reviewed the list with him, he looked very sad. "But this was supposed to be after I died! You can't give away all my things now!"

I didn't know it was so hard. I actually felt physical pain in my chest. There was no way we could explain it to him. The landlord, who had been very patient and kind, had allowed us to pay several months' rent to hold the apartment while Roger's plans were indefinite. Now he wanted it vacated if possible. Roger requested still more clothes and linens and wall hangings. We would do our best to carry out his wishes.

The hour was late when we left. With his permission we planned to attend worship services at First Mennonite Fellowship, come back, prepare our dinner, and eat together on the lower deck. He remembered it would be Mother's Day, so it had to be special.

24

A Day to Remember

Marvin is always an early riser. He is energized and ready to take on anything. How often I have wished for that stamina and zip. I seem to look through a fog for at least an hour and am far more tired than at the end of the day. I doubt that Marvin slept much at all the morning after our arrival. He had all the details planned as to how we would handle the task of the day.

Our morning devotions took us to Isaiah 41:10-13:

> Fear not, for I am with you, be not dismayed, for I am your God; I will strengthen you, I will help you, I will uphold you with my victorious right hand. (RSV)

With that assurance we were ready to meet the day in good spirits. We stopped at McDonalds for a quick breakfast and were able to find a parking space near the Shanti residence. We announced our arrival with our usual code. The doors were always locked for the protection of the residents.

An attendant welcomed us, and we eagerly went to Roger's room. We stopped in the doorway and exchanged several greetings.

"Happy Mother's Day," he said. Then, between audible sobs, he choked out, "You didn't get your roses! I tried to get someone to buy some for you but I couldn't get anyone to do it. I'm so sorry. I wanted so much for you to have some."

By then I was embracing him and he was shaking with sobs. I was deeply touched. I had told him that the thought was as great a gift as the gift itself, but he didn't agree. I assured him that his love was more precious than any earthly thing. He seemed more listless than usual and said his headache was severe. His linens and clothes were soaked from night sweats, and he looked dejected and miserable. Again, he wanted me to put on the *Dino* tape. We tried to think of cheerful and interesting things to talk about, but nothing seemed to matter.

Then it was time to leave for church. We promised to be back for dinner. Services were from ten to eleven o'clock, and we needed to be back at his apartment by two to greet his friends.

It felt so encouraging to be among God's people in shared worship and experience God's presence. We no longer were strangers among them. We gained needed strength and energy for the day.

Back at the Shanti residence I busied myself in the kitchen. How could getting a meal be so difficult? There were as many meals being prepared as there were patients and workers; pots, pans, and dishes had to be shared. It seemed to take twice as long. The menu was more abbreviated than usual. I had asked Marvin to get Roger ready, put him in the wheelchair, and take him to the deck. There was an outside walkway through a garden area to the deck.

I carried the food down the two flights of stairs while Marvin was trying to get Roger comfortable in a big lounge chair. The warm sunshine felt therapeutic and the setting was gorgeous. How much we'll enjoy this, I thought. I was wrong. I gave Roger his plate of food and, as usual, he immediately began to eat. Before I could get ours ready, he said he had to get back to bed. We encouraged him to lie back in the lounge and rest, but he couldn't stand it.

Marvin hurriedly ate a few bites and took him back to his room. I wasn't hungry, so I gathered up the food and dishes and in several trips up the rather steep and open stairway I carried everything back to the kitchen. My dress-up clothes and heels were not really designed for this! Twice during the ordeal Roger spontaneously burst out with the message that he loved us. There is much power, comfort, and joy in those few words. We have learned through his example to say them more often.

When we were ready to leave, there was searching and sadness in Roger's eyes. I thought I couldn't bear it. Silently I prayed for strength. The beautiful day made it easier. I bought some snacks and drinks for friends who would come to his old apartment.

The house was in order. Everything was pulled out and names put on things. We had been there an hour when the phone rang. We had not yet disconnected it. It was Roger. He said he wanted Dad to come and get him. I tried to reason with him that it would be too hard for him, that I didn't think it wise or helpful. He was insistent.

I finally handed the phone to Marvin. All I heard was: "Well . . . okay. I'll come and get you."

I couldn't believe it. Can Roger hold up under the pressure of giving up everything? I thought. Sometimes I wished I could simply vanish. I wasn't sure I could endure much more.

I watched from the living room windows as they drove up. Roger got out of the car with a struggle and staggered to the gate. I greeted him at the door.

He walked directly to the piano he had recently purchased, which still sat in the middle of the room. He sat down on the piano bench and, in concert style, with accuracy and energy, his fingers rippled and pounded all over the keyboard, playing the great hymn of affirmation, "Trust and Obey."

I couldn't believe my eyes and ears—I was so stunned! I knew it had come from the Lord. It was as though Roger was saying, "It's okay. That's what I'm doing."

Sandy, a fellow employee of Pacific Bell, was standing near by. Her mouth dropped open in surprise. She gasped and then exclaimed, "I can't believe it, Roger! I didn't even know you could play!"

He got from the piano bench by himself with the help of his four-footed cane, ambled over to the thermostat, and turned up the heat. Next went to the bed, pulled back the covers, and crawled in, coat, scarf, hat, and all. Then he heaved a big sigh. The rest of us all smiled. He had accomplished quite a feat!

Suddenly he looked at Sandy. "What are you doing here?"

"I came to pick up the things you wanted me to have," she said.

"Like what?"

"The picture above the dining table."

"No, you can't have that," he said emphatically. "What else?"

Slowly and reluctantly she said, "One of the art pieces by the fireplace."

"No, Sandy, not now. You can't have my things now!" He looked around. "Mom, Dad, you can't give all my things away!" His voice was shaking, his body trembling. With that, he threw back the covers, got out of bed, and muttered, "I gotta go."

Dad helped him to the outside doorway. Slowly Roger

turned around in the foyer, looked all around, hung his head, and very sadly said, "Good-bye, little house. . . ."

I thought my heart would break. As they drove away, I could see his head turned until they were out of sight.

In the car Marvin told him, "I couldn't believe what I heard. Was that Liberace playing in your house?"

"No, that was me," Roger said, pleased with himself.

"What was it that you played?" Marvin asked.

"It was 'Trust and Obey?'"

"I guess that's all we need to do."

"Yes, that's all we need to do," was Roger's reply.

Roger's simple affirmation of faith and peace was enough.

After getting him back to bed in the Shanti home he seemed relaxed. Marvin stayed and spent some time with him. Roger knew closing up his house had to be done, but it just seemed so final. He didn't know what little time was left for him. As was his pattern, he would make the most of it.

Friends came and went at the house all afternoon. It was heartwarming to meet them and listen to their comments of the special place Roger held in their hearts. His life had touched many. One by one they received his belongings. I didn't know there could be so much, for it was a collection of an entire household, including the carpet and car. Can you imagine living to see everything you every owned and cherished given away?

After all the work was finished, friends stayed to be with us for heart-to-heart talks. We heard more stories of sorrow and rejection and learning to live in a society that lacks understanding and acceptance. My heart was so full I thought it would explode. We had learned to love these friends. They showed such sensitivity in trying to make our days easier. The memory of that day will always remain.

25

Stretcher Bearers

One day seemed to blend into another. Sometimes it was difficult to remember which day it was. We came and went with the flow. There was always yet another thing to do. It was quite unlike a vacation away from home. We will be eternally grateful for those dear people who stood by us. They taught us a lot about love. I believe we received more hugs throughout Roger's illness than in a lifetime before that. We have learned how to share our love in more significant ways. They were available to run errands, do business, or just sit with Roger or us. We noticed that everyone was treated with respect and dignity, without gossip. Each was known by his/her name; it was like a big family and it felt good.

One morning we came rather early so we could make every minute count for good. As I walked back to the kitchen for a refill for Roger's pitcher, I noticed Victor's door was almost closed and the room looked dark. When I looked in, I noticed a candle burning on his dresser. The bed had been stripped. Then I knew that Victor had died during the night. I felt sad. Victor was a Haitian and had no family here. He had acquired AIDS through using IV drugs. He had no one here to help him through his difficult time.

I went to the kitchen and stood by the window that

overlooked the city. It was an awesome sight. I remembered the picture of Jesus on the mount, lamenting over Jerusalem, and felt something of his agony (Matt. 23:37).

Have I made a difference? Has my life been a flicker of light in the darkness? Probing questions pricked my heart. Slowly I made my way down the hall. As I passed Steve's room, I saw a hospice volunteer sitting by his bed tenderly rubbing his leg. No one spoke—there was just caring concern. Steve had Kaposi's sarcoma. Soon I would find his bed also stripped. Why did his family and friends reject him?

Again I was thankful for these volunteers who willingly shared of their time and love with those who needed someone. I felt such sorrow for all these dear ones. They were so young to have life snatched away while they had much to give. The suffering was incredible. If only I could do something to make someone better. One thing was sure? I would befriend anyone I knew to be friendless or needed someone to care for them. I too had love to give.

Roger had taken a painting to a shop to be framed and requested that we pick it up. Among other errands, he wanted the oil painting of Bali which had been such an inspiration to him. It was too big for our compact rented car. Mark offered to bring it in his station wagon between his work assignments that day. He would meet us at Roger's house.

As we left the Shanti residence, we met a woman coming in. She greeted us warmly with a big hug and introduced herself as Gretchen. She spoke with an accent.

"Do you have family here?" I asked.

"No, but these are my dear friends, and I come to visit them regularly."

When we told her who we were, she said, "It is so good to meet you. You are special people!" Her response was exuberant, and we knew she meant what she said.

We learned that she was wonderfully therapeutic and loved by these residents and was filling the gap for those who had no one to love them. She had taken a special interest in Victor, and was sad when she learned of his death.

One more trip to the house for incidentals would wrap it up. Roger was concerned that his many plants have a good home. Some were so large that it took several persons to carry them. Roger had no space for them. We noticed that the Shanti living room appeared sterile without any living plants, and asked the staff if plants would be accepted. Absolutely, they said.

By noon we were back with the Bali painting and three large plants with elaborate macrame hangers that Roger had made. Someone brought a plant stand for another. The living room was quite improved with the lovely plants. When we hung the painting on Roger's wall, he was so pleased.

He had wanted more dress clothes. I couldn't tell him he would never need them—and there was no room in his closet for more. I brought several outfits, and he seemed satisfied.

Since Ted wore the same size, we suggested he take the good suits, shirts, and ties. Ted agreed that at any time Roger needed them, he would be glad to get them for him. Later he came over, went through Roger's closet, and took what he wanted.

Pastor Ruth Buxman had become a daily visitor. Roger almost demanded her time and she was very generous with it. What a comfort she was to him and what a joy to us. She was truly an answer to our prayers and helped Roger through his search for forgiveness. God, in his own time and own way, brought it to pass, and Roger finally felt forgiven. During the many hours Ruth had spent with him, she helped him process his quest for peace.

Ruth and Doug were very considerate of our needs. With our consent they arranged to take us to a unique Japanese restaurant for dinner. It was a very special evening. It was so authentic that some took off their shoes and ate at low tables, sitting on the floor. But there were tables for people like us who chose not to conform to Japanese style!

The meal was served in courses, with chopsticks only. Who ever heard of eating soup with chopsticks? We were told we couldn't ask for spoons. Somehow my sticks weren't coordinated. Neither Marvin nor I were sure we would survive this meal, but Doug and Ruth tried to teach us how it was done. We laughed, had a wonderful time, and enjoyed the two-hour meal very much. For a brief interlude we were totally relaxed and relieved of the pain that never seemed to go away. We loved them so much for this deed of kindness.

When we returned to the Shanti residence, we found Roger very listless. He had had episodes of gastrointestinal problems most of the afternoon and was experiencing intense pain. I could only hold him close and tell him that I loved him. He asked me to rub his back, which I did. Dad also rubbed his feet which relaxed him.

Sometimes we talked; sometimes we just sat quietly, knowing that we were close. The hour was late, but we were reluctant to leave. I was glad that we could go home, knowing someone would be there to help him if he needed something.

His lethargy and diarrhea continued the next day. His pulse was rapid, his face flushed, his breathing shallow. His temperature climbed higher than usual, although he always had a fever even on a regular medication regimen. I encouraged more fluids, but he took only a few sips at a time. It was hard to see him suffer. He lay with his eyes closed most of the time.

As Marvin talked with Ruth on the phone, she thoughtfully asked if we would like to have communion with Roger. We would be leaving the next day and thought it was a wonderful idea. We agreed on three o'clock in the afternoon. Friends were in and out during the day, and it seemed we were never alone; and I was afraid we would have to ask for the special time.

When the time was appropriate, she brought in the bread and juice. She explained our desire to Roger and related the purpose of communion.

"Do you understand it was because Jesus died for our sins to make it possible that we could have life forever with him in heaven? We want to remember what he did for us." she spoke slowly and carefully.

He nodded. "Yes, I do."

Marvin, Ruth, and I took turns reading Psalm 103. Never did it hold so much meaning for me as it did now! Ruth prayed, then offered the elements to each of us. It was a sacred moment to share together. I felt the presence of Jesus in that room. After the final prayer, we held each other and let the tears flow. I think it was my final act of completely releasing Roger to the Lord.

He appeared completely at rest. Without another word, he fell into a deep sleep.

We would be leaving in the morning. I dreaded to go, for the need to engage in any kind of meaningful conversation was now over. He had found forgiveness and was ready for a better world; he had suffered enough. But how we would miss him! I wished so much he could have experienced what should have been the best part of his life.

I called Peggy, the hospice nurse, to check on his

deteriorating condition. I asked all the unanswerable questions: Is there any way you can predict how much longer he has? If you have a clue, would you please call us? She assured us that she would call if there could be prediction. If possible, we wanted to be with him when he died.

Earlier in the week, we had made an appointment with the mortuary, legal papers had been signed, and final arrangements made. It probably was the most difficult thing we had ever done, but it needed to be taken care of in case we were not there.

All that was left to do was to say good-bye. "Maybe we'll be back soon," I told him.

He nodded his head and whispered, "I love you. . . ."

26

The Last Farewell

We arrived home on Friday morning. Sheryl and Leo picked us up at the airport, eager for all the details. It felt good to be home, but my mind was not at rest. Perhaps we should've stayed. How many times we thought it would be the last time! Both of us were tired enough to sleep that night.

The next morning I was expecting the usual morning call, but it didn't come. About midafternoon I decided to call. What a pleasant surprise to hear Derek's voice. Roger had liked him so well as a hospice nurse when he was still in his home. Now he worked weekends at the Shanti residence to fill in for someone who was ill.

"Helen, things are not good," he said gravely. "I put him on oxygen. He's having a lot of trouble breathing. His bowels are giving him problems and he is incontinent. He's a very sick guy."

I told Derek that I was relieved he was there. I knew that he was in good hands and I could rest much easier. I also knew that Roger was most comfortable with him. He thanked me for the confidence but warned me about the possibility of a call.

I knew our calls from Roger were over. On Sunday afternoon I called back so that I could talk to Derek. The report was no better. Roger was very sick. Monday afternoon's call was no different. His condition was critical, the attendant reported. I urged him to keep in touch.

Tuesday evening the expected call came. "Hello, Helen." I knew it was Peggy's voice. My heart was pounding in my throat.

"You'd better come right away," she said. "I started him on the morphine regimen. His breathing is very labored. I don't think he'll last long."

I groped for words. "We probably can't leave until the early morning flight. Do you think he'll make it until then?" I was trembling and the phone receiver shook in my hands.

"I can't tell you. He is very, very sick and you'd better come as soon as you can. Just in case you don't get here, we have rigged up an extension that we hope will work, so you can talk to him," she added.

I waited anxiously for his voice. It was ragged.

"Mom . . . I love you . . . hurry and . . . come. I'm dying. Please come as soon as you . . . can." There was such urgency in his crying voice. I assured him would get there as soon as possible. I knew it would probably be 1:15 p.m. on Wednesday before we could get there.

"Please . . . hurry!" he said again.

"We love you and will see you soon," was all I could say.

I thanked Peggy for calling and quickly told Marvin, who was in the backyard.

He was able to get plane tickets and cash. I had kept the laundry done daily, so it didn't take me long to put a few things together. We would need fewer clothes on this trip.

I called the girls, family, a few close friends, and our pastor. An amazing calm surrounded us, and we were able to go to bed and sleep. Sheryl and Leo again took us to the plane early in the morning. It's hard to express the peace we had as we lifted above the clouds and headed for Phoenix. The familiar words of P. P. Bliss came to mind:

> When peace, like a river, attendeth my way,
> When sorrows like sea billows roll;
> Whatever my lot, thou hast taught me to say,
> It is well, it is well with my soul.

During the two-hour layover in Phoenix we went for a walk in the warm sunshine. It was as though God was smiling on us, giving us his warmth. The other plane passengers were oblivious to what we were feeling.

Our plane landed in Oakland on schedule. Being familiar with procedures by now, we hurried over to the car rental and picked up our car. It was noon, but we decided not to take time for anything to eat. Marvin wove in and out of the heavy traffic like a pro and we felt more relaxed, knowing the road and its exits.

At exactly 1:15 p.m. we parked our car a block from the Shanti residence. We rang our usual code with the door bell. Six of Roger's friends greeted us at the door. Another woman introduced herself as Dale's mother. Dale lived across the hall from Roger. I was surprised to see her, as Dale's parents lived in a distant small town. The presence of AIDS within their community was not even remotely considered. They lived in loneliness and fear of their family secret leaking out. The father had been unable to deal with the fact of his son's dying and, of all things, with AIDS! The mother took courage and determined to visit her son. We only briefly shared our pilgrimage with her in the hope that she might be encouraged. I am sorry that we had no further contact with her.

They said Roger was anxious to see us, and we made

our way to his room. I wasn't prepared for what I saw. He was packed in ice, was getting oxygen, and his breathing was very labored. His eyes were glassy and I hardly recognized him.

When he saw us he let out a feeble yell and stretched out his arms. "I'm . . . dying," he whispered.

"It's okay," I said as we embraced for a long time.

"I'm *so* glad . . . you're here." his voice cracked.

It was his dad's turn for a tearful hug. Ruth and Rosemary were with him in the room while others waited in the living room. I pulled a chair next to the bed, and Dad sat on the bed on the other side. Roger was struggling for every breath he took and it was difficult for his father to watch. From time to time he left the room.

Roger reached up his arms and said, "Give me . . . another . . . hug, Mom. . . ." He was burning hot in spite of the ice packs.

The nurses were in and out frequently, monitoring the equipment. I repeated the 23rd Psalm close to his ear and turned his well-loved *Dino* tape on softly,

"You look . . . so nice, Mom. That's a . . . pretty blouse." It was such a struggle to talk.

"Are you ready to see Jesus?" I asked.

He nodded. "I'm so glad . . . you're here," he repeated again and again. He glanced at Ruth, who was seated on the love seat, and said, "Ruth, you can leave . . . if you need to."

"Okay, Roger," she said, but she stayed.

I repeated a number of Bible promises to him! "Let not your heart be troubled. . . . There are many rooms in my Father's house and I'm going to prepare them for your coming. . . . Peace I leave with you. . . . Let not your heart be troubled, neither let it be afraid."

"Roger, there is laid up for you a crown of righteousness! We shall all be given new bodies . . . just think, a brand-new perfect body that can never be sick again!"

Eight friends stayed throughout the evening. His breathing grew less labored, more shallow. Once he looked up at me with searching eyes, and said, "You won't forget me, will you?" How could he think that we could ever forget him?

Frequently he whispered, "I love you. . . ." His eyes were closed now, and his position changed every two hours. Marvin was in and out of the room. It was too hard to watch his son die by inches.

By now it was evening. We had not eaten since early morning. I was concerned about Marvin, who is a diabetic and needed to eat regularly.

Ruth and Doug insisted we get a sandwich or something to eat. I hated to go, but everyone encouraged us to leave for a brief time. They took us to a small restaurant a short distance away. It was refreshing to get away for a little while.

Our pastor had called while we were gone, and so had Sheryl. We were sorry to have missed them.

Roger's respirations were shallow. I wondered how long it could continue.

One of Roger's friends, seated on the bed near me, put his arms around me and whispered, "What can I do for you? I just feel so sad and helpless." That was comfort.

About 1:00 a.m. I noticed that Roger's breathing pattern had changed to gasping, and I knew the end was near. His pulse was thready . . . then imperceptible. I asked Rosemary to get Marvin, who was in the other room. The six friends who had stayed also came in. We all watched as Roger's breathing became less—and then he took his last breath. His spirit had crossed over to the other world.

One by one his friends told him good-bye. I stood frozen beside the body of my son.

"The Lord has given. The Lord has taken away. Blessed be the name of the Lord," I choked out between sobs.

His long journey was over. Peace at last! I had given him the last hug. We had loved him to the end. He was now in the arms of his heavenly Father. He looked so handsome at rest, when all the paraphernalia was removed, and the nurses quietly left.

For thirty minutes we lingered in his room. Weakly I walked to the love seat and sat down. Ruth came and sat beside me.

"He looks so special," she whispered, her arms around my shoulders. "Do you see the face of Jesus?"

What a beautiful observation! She could have offered no greater comfort. I too believed it.

> I have fought a good fight,
> I have finished my course,
> I have kept the faith: Henceforth there is laid up for me
> a crown of righteousness, which the Lord, the righteous
> judge, shall give me at that day. (2 Timothy 4:7-8)

The charge nurse came in to ask if we needed more time. We had enough, and got up to leave. I turned for a last look at my dear son. How peaceful he looked!

In the hallway stood the mortician. Chills raced up and down my spine as I realized the finality of it all. With legs that felt wooden, I started for the door.

27

Time for Tribute

Before leaving for the motel we made arrangements to meet at Jeff's apartment, along with his close friends, for brunch at ten o'clock in the morning. We would plan details for Roger's memorial service to carry out his wishes.

The night was chilly and damp; low, forbidding clouds hung low over the horizon as we headed back to our motel near the bay. Honking horns from the tugboat blared in the distance. For the first time we were not fighting traffic. As we made our final exit, we discovered they were resurfacing the street. Marvin accepted the challenge and crossed the median to the other side and proceeded down the tar-drenched roadway. I gasped as I heard the rain and clatter of tar and small gravel on the lower surface of our car. The road crew looked up with dismay as we edged our way out of the construction area. We looked at each other and chuckled. Had we chosen to comply with the detour we would certainly have been lost.

As we walked toward our motel room, which was located to the back overlooking the bay, we could see a million lights reflected on the water and hear the waves lapping on the shore. We heard the swish and swoop of sea gulls on the cliffs. There we stood in awe, almost numb. Was it really over? We still couldn't grasp it all.

We made numerous phone calls to family and friends. Roger had requested that Bob be in charge of the service in San Francisco. Bob and Linda were special friends from college days. He was now a pastor in Ojai, California. Roger had spent holidays with them, and their two daughters were darlings. We would call them in the morning.

It was now 3:15, but sleep didn't come. There was a real sense of peace, yet deep sorrow at our loss. In the days to come we would begin to make some sense of it all. We would come to understand the meaning of the prophecy Betty gave concerning Roger.

The following morning we met at Jeff's along with six other friends. Around his table we reflected on Roger's life and his love and influence on us. It was an intense time of sharing the memory which we will always hold close to our hearts. Again, it was miraculous how information and plans all fused together. Jan, a dear friend who had played a significant role in the days of his illness, had traveled to Canada to dispose of property and finalize plans for a permanent residence in San Francisco. We did not know how she could be reached and placed a telephone call to her vacated house. She had returned just at that moment on an errand and picked up her telephone. How grateful we all were to have contacted her! Bob's weekend schedule also was full except for the day chosen for the service. It was incredible how people were notified and responsibilities assumed. We know one thing for certain: God was in control.

Roger had requested cremation and wished to be buried beside our burial site in McPherson. We had to make arrangements at the mortuary to be able to take his cremains home with us for a service that was to be held in McPherson for relatives and friends at home.

What would we do for a day and a half? We determined to get a glimpse of the beauty of this city, which had often been shrouded by a cloud in our earlier visits. We sat by the ocean that Roger loved, listened to the roar of sea lions and scream of gulls, watched the ships, and gazed at the endless horizon.

The awesomeness of it all was moving. We were able to gather strength as we experienced the Lord's presence with us. Leisurely we visited Louie's by the Cliff House and ate prawns. We watched the waves lap and surge on the cliff directly below us.

We drove through Golden Gate Park to Stowe Lake, the spot of our last picnic with Roger. We paused and meditated as we watched a family feed bread to the pigeons. We visited the beautiful arboretum, museum, Hall of Flowers, and remembered how much joy this had given Roger. We saw the intricate Victorian architecture in the residential area. The well-preserved hand-painted artistic gingerbread intrigued us. The quaint streetcars caught our attention as they clanked and clanged up and down the hilly streets. We climbed the twin peaks for a last glimpse of the city with Alcatraz and Golden Gate Bridge in the background. It was impressive. We visited the zoo and marveled at the expanse of natural habitat that had been created for the animals.

Tickets were confirmed for our return flight home, and we would leave immediately after the 10:30 a.m. service on Friday, May 23, 1986. It was to be conducted in the graceful sanctuary of the Unitarian Church in downtown San Francisco.

Bob would be in charge of the service. Approximately fifty friends attended. Taped selections from the Gay Men's Chorus, of which he had been a part, drifted softly over the quiet background. Taken from the taped service, the following remarks and tributes were given:

Bob: "Jesus said, I am the resurrection and I am Life. Those who believe in me, even though they may die, Yet shall they live. Whosoever lives and believes in me shall never die. I am Alpha and Omega—the beginning and the end, the first and the last. Because I live—you shall live also. I hold the keys to eternity."

Friends, we are together in this place, with each other, to praise God and to witness our faith and our love, as we celebrate the life of Roger Hostetler. We came together acknowledging our grief, knowing our sorrow, and we ask in the presence of God and each other that our hearts may be searched, and that in our pain we may find comfort, in our sorrow we may find hope, and in the face of death we may know the certain promise of resurrection.

Opening Prayer: Almighty God, you gave us birth. You are ever more ready to come to us and to hear our needs than we are even to ask them. We ask now that you would give us your grace, that as we shrink before the mystery of death, we may know the certain light of eternity. Help us, O God, to live as those who are prepared to die, and when our summons comes, may we die as those who go forth to live. So that in our living or our dying, our life may be in you and nothing in life or death will be able to separate us from your great love. Amen.

Bob: Roger Oliver Hostetler was born in McPherson, Kansas, May 4, 1950. He died May 21, 1986, in San Francisco, California. We are here this day to worship in reverence and faith in memory of Roger, who at the age of 36 passed away to be with God on Wednesday morning. Death didn't come unexpectedly. Roger was the victim of an unrelenting, progressive disease that finally claimed him. In his weakening and deteriorating state, it is almost as if Roger saw an opening and he took it.

Roger was not afraid of death, not happy about it, yet not panicky in the face of death. He said he would be happy finally to be at peace and to leave the suffering of the body he had experienced in these later months, also to leave the suffering he had seen on this planet. He believed that in the afterlife there would be a place of bliss where there was no suffering, and Roger claimed that promise. He is at peace. But even still, his passing is to us a shock, and we as family and friends have difficulty in accepting it.

In the land of Bali that Roger visited, for which he grew to have great fondness, the death ceremony is a celebration; and it was indeed Roger's expressed wish that this memorial service be in that very nature. Well, perhaps we can. It's not easy, but in the presence of each other and with the music of the Gay Men's Chorus in our ears we can celebrate. We can celebrate the life of Roger; we can celebrate the blessings he left with us and the memories we will always cherish. We will try to do that.

Some 15 years ago Roger drove his friend Lynda Schrock down a dusty, gravel road in Indiana and ended up on the paved streets of Boston. It was there that I first met Roger and I came to know him as a friend who would do far more than drive another friend 1,000 miles. And so when Lynda and I were married, Roger was there with his guitar. He sang at our wedding. And when we had given birth to our girls, Roger was there to welcome them into the life of the world. He became important to them in their infancy, their toddler period, and also early elementary school age. Roger would pick them up, and in turn they and their spirits and appreciation for him picked up on Roger. He became part of our family, and he sometimes would refer to us as his other family. We so enjoyed his presence.

I can remember so many things: his showing up at the front door with gifts under his arms, a generous smile on his face that could so readily blossom into a pitched laugh. The music that he would pound out on the piano, or even pound out with his tap shoes. The delightful aroma of food that Roger would bring to the kitchen, and we could enjoy the food that he cooked and he enjoyed so much. The very subtle hint of satisfaction that I picked up from Roger's characteristic flicking of his fingers, and I know that Roger was comfortable. And then the many heartfelt conversations that we had after meals that would go long into the evening. I remember, too, the excitement of being in Roger's home and feeling like I was a loved one and he was treating us like a loved one. He would treat us to those things which he himself enjoyed so much. We could enjoy a musical, a symphony, a museum, a picnic in the park. Roger had an exceptional appreciation for beauty and the things of life that were eternal, and he seemed to be very comfortable without those temporal things in life that give no lasting meaning.

Music was part of his life. The music we hear today is part of the selections he enjoyed so much. He selected these pieces for us. Roger also had a great fondness for art and for the natural world of nature. He was a bright, warm, creative, and energetic person and he was not shackled by superficial things that so easily become pressing in our lives. Roger was a free-spirited person. He was a certain blessing to be around, sharing that spirit. And now Roger has inherited all those things which are eternal.

Roger had asked that his dad and I share some words with his friends. How could we, I wondered? We wanted to carry out his wishes, so we did our best. Here's what we said:

Mom: How does a mother give a fitting tribute to a son who was loved so much—and had so much love to give? Roger was a real part of us. He was conceived in love, dedicated to God, and given back to God again. His happiness and disappointments were ours. His achievements and aspirations also belonged to us. I recall watching him as a toddler reach for a sunbeam—and chase butterflies, stopping in disappointment as they went out of sight.

He had a generous and compassionate heart toward the hurting, the disadvantaged, the lonely, and the handicapped. There were few brother-sister fights. Many things come to mind as I reminisce about his childhood. I remember the day that Janene's pet dog darted into the street and was run over by an approaching car, and the anguished cries that we heard as she stopped to pick up her very cherished friend, now dead. I saw Roger rush to her, trying to console her, wrapping her in his arms, offering to carry her dog against resistance—his arms around her and tears also running down his cheeks. He too was very sad.

He demonstrated much courage and strength in the days of his illness. He faced death with confidence, assurance, and peace. Early in his youth he made a choice that determined his eternal destiny. The words of our Lord gave much comfort, "I am leaving you with a gift—peace of mind and heart. And the peace I give isn't fragile like the peace the world gives, so don't be troubled and don't be afraid" (John 14:27).

The rainbow he put into our lives will continue to live on, literally and symbolically. The stained-glass art pieces and crystals, that many of you have now to treasure, are symbolic. Away from the sunlight, they are dull and drab, even appearing dark. Put them where the sun shines through them and they are brilliant in color, casting rainbows everywhere. I like to think that allowing the Son, Jesus himself, to shine through us, puts beauty and brilliance into our lives wherever we go.

Roger's love for beauty, music, peace, and harmony is now complete in that eternal dwelling place. Our joy will also be complete when we can again be reunited. Thank you, Roger, for your greatest gift to us, the gift of your love.

Dad: My friends back home would never believe it if they knew that I was telling you that I am almost without words! But if I can't get any farther, I really want to say that I totally agree with what his mother has said. Rather than go back into his life, I would like to tell you of some observations I made here in San Francisco. Yesterday we went out to Stowe Lake. There was a young lady feeding the pigeons with some bread that didn't look very good. She was breaking off pieces and throwing them out to the pigeons. Her husband was there watching and he said somehow or other the yeast or leaven didn't work right and the bread was no good. This morning I'd like to look at you as a loaf of bread. And I think that because Roger was the leaven that entered your lives, you are much better people than if he had never met you.

That's a homely little expression but I have a little book here—it's not nearly as big as Bob's, but it has the same New Testament in it. It talks about leaven. Jesus taught with parables. Maybe what I'm telling you can be a little parable. But Jesus was saying there was a woman who had some leaven and she hid it in a lump of meal until it all became leaven. I think I see faces here that I consider very dear friends of mine; I love you, and the God that loved Roger loves you too, and if you want the peace he had, all you need to do, regardless whether you are as imperfect as I am—I make mistakes all the time—is to ask God for that peace—it's yours.

Lynda: I feel honored to be identified by Roger as his "other family." It was Roger's wish that our entire family be here. Bob and I are, but Rebecca who is eight and Laura, five, are not here today. On their behalf I want to tell you that Roger meant a great deal to them in their lives, and it is evidenced by the name they gave him. They call him "Uncle Roger." For me, he was a brother and friend of long standing. We were carefree college students together back in 1968. I really appreciate the enduring quality of our friendship over these years. Roger was a tenacious friend. He worked hard and made sure that we had continued contact. It was always a meaningful contact, not superficial. It endured the miles and the years over this period of time. I'll always consider him a true and forever friend.

Another aspect of our friendship that I so much appreciate about Roger is that he taught me a lot by the way in which he related to people as a nurturing and caring person. He cared for living things. He cared about his plants and he made then thrive; he cared about living people and he made *them* thrive.

In Boston, at one point, he had a position in the State Institution, Fernalds, where he did custodial care. He would describe to me these persons that he took care of, and I came to know them as real persons. Then one day he took Bob and me to meet his friends, his clients, his patients, and I was so startled because they seemed so incapable of being loved, so repulsive, and it seemed so difficult for me to see them as people. And yet, Roger affirmed their personhood, even though they were rejects, institutionalized for life. So that's something that I'll always remember about Roger. He was always affirming of everyone and he always affirmed me.

Another thing I have really liked about my relationship with Roger over the years is that he had a unique ability to enjoy the pleasures of life, and that's already been alluded to by other people. For example, a good meal. We shared many good laughs and many mundane moments too, as well as outings, trips, little vacations together, and experiences in nature. I want to read briefly from Henry

David Thoreau's *Walden's*, because when we both were in
Boston we would go to Walden's Pond; picnic, hike, and
such. Thoreau is describing living deliberately and
pleasurably each day—which is exactly how I feel that
Roger lived his life. Thoreau says:

> Time is but the stream I go a-fishing in
> I drink at it, but while I drink, I see the sandy bottom
>   and detect how shallow it is.
> Its thin currents slide away
> but eternity remains.
> I would drink deeper, fish in the sky whose bottom is
>   pebbly with stars.
> I cannot count one. Eternity remains.

My feeling today is that of affirmation, that Roger is
enjoying, experiencing fully that eternity as he did those
simple pleasures of life that I was privileged to share with
him. I feel that I have been given a gift from God to have
participated in his life and death.

Jan: I assume that Roger's spirit is here and enjoying
the white roses in the black vase and the scarf from Bali.
I want to also acknowledge Annie's presence here. I want
to say a little bit of what I think she might have said. She
was a real sister of Roger's and gave unstintingly of her
love, as did several others. It's been of value in my life to
have spent this past year knowing Roger, and to discover
a new aspect of love that I had not known quite so well
before—that of giving. I felt like I came into Roger's life in
a rather strange sort of way and experienced giving to
him a lot. And I also experienced his giving of himself
through the cloud of his illness in a way that was really
enlivening for me, and for the rest of you, I'm sure.

Ted: I am also a little Kansas farm boy, and I think
that attracted me to Roger when I first saw him in the
SFGMC (San Francisco Gay Men's Chorus). We became

seatmates and we sometimes stood in the back and watched, wondering whether it was really all right that we were singing in the SFGMC. We shared the rehearsals and the afterglows. I think one of the most confusing and frustrating, yet most rewarding and questioning times of our lives was the tour. That experience exemplified the closeness that we had, and somehow I feel a lot of Roger's spirit in me, as I question life and enjoy and discover who I am. I feel that in dying Roger gave me a gift that he could never have given me by living: letting me know his parents. I have found myself drawn to the words of one of the songs that we did on tour. I will try to sing it for you: "'Tis the gift to be simple, 'Tis the gift to be free. . . ."

Rosemary: I'm glad we're all here—that Roger gave us this so that we could all be together today. When Roger was planning his memorial, he told me that he would like for me to say something. I felt already that this was going to be hard. I said, "What shall I say?" and he said, "Just say that you were my friend and you loved me." I was his friend and I loved him. He was like my soul mate in life.

It really was Roger's wish that he make a contribution, and we know that he certainly did. He contributed to each of us in a special way. Last year when he was quite sick, he said to me, "Well, maybe through my going through this will change your life, will have an effect on you, and it will be good." For a long time I really resisted that; I was not going to give him that. Somehow I just didn't want to do that. He was right. He absolutely changed my life. I have softened a whole lot—and surrendered. It's going to affect the way I live my life, having been through this with him and being with him. I have never been with anyone who has died before. Being with him when he died was a very intimate experience.

Mark: I have heard so much about Roger giving in his life, and it was so true with me. I remember feeling through our relationship in that I was walking away, always feeling that I was the one receiving. It seemed that it should have been the other way. With time I grew to know that it was natural and was Roger's way. In that way Roger touched me, and I'm very grateful.

Jeff: Shanti became the vehicle through which I met Roger. As many of you know, Roger developed a very special attachment to me which became overwhelming to me at times because I came to him through a volunteer contract. It's taken me a long time to sort out what our relationship meant. I think one thing that he would want me to share is the love he had for me and sometimes feeling awkward I could not return it to him. On Monday night we shared a very special time together. He was always concerned about making a contribution in this world before he left to make his transition. The contribution he made to me Monday night was allowing me to lie next to him and say to him, "I love you," and say it from the heart, not allowing my mind to get in the way. I think we so oftimes are put in situations that allow our minds to get in the way of sharing and telling people that we love them, and we hold back from that. Now is the time to do that and there is time to love. In thinking about what I wanted to share, I don't often read but I would like to share from one of the great philosophers in the Bible: [He read from 1 Corinthians 13.] I love you, Roger.

Pastor Ruth Buxman from First Mennonite Fellowship pronounced the benediction, and the service closed with the beautiful *Allelulia* from Wagner.

Silently we sat in our pews weeping, then one by one we shared greetings of love. The white roses were passed out to Roger's closest friends. There were no words that could adequately convey the message of love and thanksgiving we felt for those who had so uniquely and unselfishly touched our lives. We could never forget them. God would reward them. Good-byes seemed so final.

Our bags were packed in the car, and we had to hurry away for a noon flight out of Oakland. We took a last look at this city which had played such a significant role in our lives.

28

Blessed Be Sorrow

Unlike our usual flight plan which took us through Phoenix, we were ticketed through Denver. Of all the airports I have been in, none were so jammed with passengers. Not only were people sitting on their luggage and lying on the floor but packed arm to arm in standing-room-only areas. Passengers whose flights were delayed or canceled, were angry; children cried; the air was stifling with cigarette smoke. Planes were lined up on the runways waiting the all-clear for takeoff.

We were carrying the white roses from Ted. It was such a lovely gesture. We also had some from the service. In our carryon bag was our precious cargo, Roger's cremains, that we guarded very carefully. We were standing by the windows where people were deplaning, but mostly we were gazing out into space.

One gentleman from the far side came and offered seats to us. Maybe we were not hiding our emotions as well as we thought. We graciously accepted and were relieved to sit down.

Finally our departure was announced. We were eager to board our plane for that last stretch home. So much was behind us, and we relaxed. We had plans to make when we got home. Tomorrow was soon enough to think of that.

Sheryl and Leo met us in Wichita. It was good to feel their arms around us. How faithful they had been! The bond of love is sweet and strong. Janene had promised to come early in the morning since driving the distance to Salina alone late at night was not wise.

Neighbors, friends, and relatives had prepared lunch for our arrival. The story would be shared again, and again, and again. What a comfort are family and friends!

After a night of sleep, we would plan for a memorial service at home. Family from Colorado and Indiana came to be with us. The days through which we had just passed and the days that lay immediately ahead were probably among the most difficult in our lives.

As we went to bed, I tried to think of all the things for which I could be thankful. They ticked through my mind like a tape recorder: for the intimacies cherished with Roger and for the times we were privileged to spend together; for the love we shared and knowing that God loves all of us far more than we can understand; for the lessons learned, the good accomplished, the influence for good that will linger on and on because of the witness that we left with them. I am thankful for our faith and the faith of others who walked this journey with us. It stood the test and God honored it. I am thankful for our home eternal, prepared for those who love God and trust him. I am thankful for hope which rules our hearts and doesn't know defeat. I am thankful for the many who sustained us and Roger with their prayers, which brought deliverance and peace. I am thankful for little associations from which we will probably never be able to fully separate ourselves: a beautiful sunset . . . a quiet lake . . . a fragrant garden of flowers . . . strains of organ music . . . the sound of a trumpet . . . family gatherings . . . holidays . . . all silent reminders of the days we spent together. Mostly, I am thankful to God, who is all-wise, all-loving, who makes no mistakes and works out his will in his own time and his own way. Praise be to God!

We arranged a service of celebration for May 27. The committal would be held at 2:00 p.m., followed by a worship service at 2:30 at First Mennonite Church of McPherson. It was planned in keeping with Roger's wishes. Since music was always a vital part of his life, we chose to use it to celebrate his life. Organ, trumpet, solo, and octet provided appropriate musical selections.

Pastor Ed R. Stucky gave the meditation, and several close friends gave tributes.

Ruby Brown: I just wanted to talk a bit about what kind of guy I knew Roger to be. I first knew him when we were about 12 or 13 years old and our fathers served on the board of the Kansas City Children's Home. I remember we went out to their farm and we met Roger there. Then we went to Goshen College together and ran around with the same group of friends. What I remember about Roger is how friendly he was. I want to give an example of that true test of friendliness that I experienced from him. Going from Goshen, Indiana, to Hesston, Kansas, is about a 17-hour trip if you stop to eat. So with six people in one car driving for 17 hours—and most cars weren't in very good shape anyway—it tested people's feelings about each other. By the time we got to Hesston at five o'clock in the morning most of us were griping at each other. Sometimes people couldn't remember where their relatives lived, so we had to drive around. Roger was the only one who would help unload luggage. Most of us were angry and upset, but Roger was still friends with all of us.

During one of those years, there was a popular song we liked. As you know, Roger was a good singer, and we thought he could sing it as well as a professional; so every once in awhile he'd humor us and sing that song. Roger had a good sense of humor, and we laughed a lot when we'd get together as friends. I think that often people who are clever and witty are also very honest; he could say things that the rest of us think but wouldn't venture to say. Roger would often be the one who would keep us laughing. Roger also liked good food. I remember one summer we visited him in Boston and he took us to a place and we had steamed clams. I haven't had any that good since.

Roger was very generous. As I was thinking about this talk I was thinking that I still owed him money. He was generous with his financial assets, with his possessions, and with his time. While he was in San Francisco he worked, or maybe owned, a company where they made silk-screened T-shirts, and I remember getting a T-shirt every three months or so. In coming here today, I knew that this was Roger's funeral, but for some reason I expected him to be here. It's very difficult to go through this with him not being here to talk about things. I want to say to his family that I'll miss him very much.

Jim: We lived within a mile of each other for more than 18 years, and that was part of the reason that Roger and I and our families were so close. It seemed that Roger and I were always together. I was told that Roger and I played together before he or I could remember. I have many fond and some not-so-fond memories of Roger. Like the time we were playing in the sandpile and were teasing the dog and I got bit! It was after this that we experienced our first day at Plainview Grade School. There were three girls and two boys in our class. Roger and I were all decked out in our new homemade shirts and jeans that were rolled up two or three notches; they just didn't make jeans short enough!

Memories prevail. Many times our parents sent us off on a trip to Rocky Mountain Mennonite Camp, in Divide, Colorado. They always said it would do us good once we got there; in looking back, they were right. We always came back with new experiences and memories to talk about. Finally the big day came in May when Roger and I and our classmates reached a milestone in our lives with eighth-grade graduation. Then it was on to Inman High School for the next four years. It's no telling how many trips we made back and forth to that town in those four years, some of which were completely necessary! I know we did our best to think of a reason to drive instead of riding that bus; then one would call and offer the other one a ride!

After high school Roger and I split ways. He went to Hesston College, then on to Goshen College, and I went here to McPherson College. No matter where we were we seemed to always call or look the other one up when we were home on holidays.

It was in March of this year that Roger contacted me and asked if there was any way that I could come out and visit him. I made arrangements and flew out the next morning. I found Roger in really good spirits. I was intrigued that he was interested in what I was doing. He reached for an envelope full of old pictures and said he would like to go through pictures from grade school and high school, just things we naturally had forgotten—and we laughed over them. When we were finished, he said, "Here, I want you to have these." The memory of that short time we spent together will be cherished throughout the remainder of my life.

In reflecting on Roger's spiritual renewal and desiring to share some encouraging words. I would like to offer the following poem written by Fanny Crosby:

Safe in the arms of Jesus, safe on his gentle breast,
There by his love o'er shaded, Sweetly my soul shall rest. . . .

Safe in the fields of glory, safe from corroding care,
Safe from the world's temptation, sin cannot harm me there.
Free from the blight of sorrow, free from my doubts and fears;
Only a few more trials, only a few more tears. . . .

Jesus my heart's dear refuge, Jesus has died for me,
Firm on the rock of ages, ever my trust shall be . . .
[and the rest of the hymn].

Jane: Roger was my cousin and when we would come from Indiana to see Marvins, Roger and I usually spent time together while my sister and Janene were together. Sheryl was too old for us. I always looked forward to being with Roger. I felt like we had so much in common, and we cared a lot about the same things. One of my most favorite memories is sitting on the grass, playing guitar, and singing. A couple of months ago I was looking through my songbook and found some songs that he wrote out for me, so I have that to keep from Roger. I also wanted to say that in the times we talked on the telephone when he was sick, the most important thing to me was that he said he was *safe in Jesus!* For a long time I had a feeling of peace that Roger would be with Jesus. Today I know that he is—and I look forward to sitting on the grass in glory with Roger!

29

Epilogue:
A Time to Love

We have allowed you to invade the privacy of our lives and have candidly shared our experiences through these pages. There have been multiple and varied gains and losses generated in our life because of Roger's AIDS. We have shared our story so that it might become a resource for a compassionate response to those who are suffering and for their families and friends. The decision to either reject or give support gravely affects the way that people with AIDS cope with their medical crises.

In telling our story, we have allowed you to observe our ignorance of the homosexuality issue and its far-reaching effect on our lives and that of our son. We have experienced the power of reaching out in love that breaks down barriers and helps to build bridges of understanding and growth.

AIDS remains a fatal disease. Several vaccines are being tested in human beings, but no one knows when a successful vaccine will be found.

The church should be a redemptive community, yet so many persons (known by the church) are abandoned, condemned, and left to die in the company of strangers. Where is the healing, the forgiveness, and the love which is professed?

I believe that people have often responded out of fear.

There is fear of transmitting this disease. It is well to remember that you cannot get AIDS through casual contact. It is not an airborne virus. It cannot live outside the human body. Family living with one who has AIDS can continue as usual: hugging, kissing, eating, and swimming together. Such relationships do not allow transmission of the virus.

Jesus commanded his fellow servants to do for one another what he had done for them. The biblical imperatives directing the church to the stranger, the outcast, and the poor are well understood and verbally accepted. Why then has the church not been more involved in ministry to those suffering with this dreadful disease?

Our story is one that, in the midst of tragedy, comfort and peace were available, and we found them. We found courage through compassionate, loving, caring relationships that spoke of the presence of God within the lives of people, those who walked with us in pain. Let those who suffer know that you care. It takes only a few words: "I don't know how you feel, but I want you to know that I care." No words are needed when there is a genuine hug. Sometimes just to be willing to listen is all that is needed; some sufferers may just be bursting to say what they feel. They will find comfort if they are not condemned and judged.

I encourage you to be informed. Much free, reliable information is available through your public health agency, the Red Cross, the Center for Disease Control in Atlanta, and the Surgeon General's reports. It is important that children are taught about family life and sexuality. Encourage openness and honesty.

It is helpful to pray publicly for those who have AIDS and for their families. It is freeing to share your pain with others who will walk this journey with you, and with those who believe in the power of prayer. It allows others to grow as they experience this difficult time with you. It also gives opportunity to bring healing for others who may be silent-sufferers. It may free someone to seek your counsel.

You can provide practical help to families who are caring for a loved one with AIDS. Laundry, cleaning, grocery shopping, and running errands are always a part of every such household. To give respite-care for a few hours is of tremendous help to these families.

Fears partly account for what appears as indifference and insensitivity, even isolation and rejection. These terrors might be overcome by courage and compassion that comes from divine love. First John 4:18-21 calls us to respond:

> There is no fear in love. But perfect love drives out fear, because fear has to do with punishment. The one who fears is not made perfect in love.

> We love because he first loved us. If anyone says, "I love God," yet hates his brother, he is a liar. For anyone who does not love his brother, whom he has seen, cannot love God, whom he has not seen. And he has given us this command: Whoever loves God must also love his brother.

Those affected by this dreaded disease must be loved with the same unmeasured love that Jesus gave. That kind of love will produce passionate ministries. The ill are people with feelings, needs, homes, and dreams. They are sons, daughters, sisters, and brothers who are suffering and dying because of a virus that destroys the body's capacity to defend itself. The suffering and grief associated with any fatal illness are compounded in the case of AIDS because of the stigmas attached to the disease. We have heard countless stories of people with AIDS who were rejected by their families and left to die among strangers. Where are the expressions of care and compassion among people who claim to give moral and spiritual leadership?

Jesus offered friendship to those who were social outcasts or considered unclean. He healed persons who had leprosy (Luke 17). The early church followed his example. Bishop Dionysius, in his letter to the Alexandrians, told how in the third century Christians tended those with the plague, at serious risk to their own lives. The pagans, however, thrust aside those who showed symptoms of plague, even their dearest friends, and cast sufferers upon public roads.

The AIDS virus (HIV, human immunodeficiency virus) is spread by sexual intercourse with an infected person, exchange of blood or blood products from an infected person, or by an infected mother to her unborn child. Caring for someone with AIDS is not as risky as helping victims of the plague.

A task force on AIDS, under Mennonite Central Committee Canada, reported: "The AIDS crisis is a challenge to the church to model the character of Jesus Christ. Our witness is at stake. We need to stop asking why people get AIDS and ask ourselves what God is calling us to."

At this writing, it is conservatively estimated that about two million persons have been infected with the AIDS virus and projections are that the number will continue to increase rapidly. It is mind-boggling to imagine the magnitude of potential suffering caused by this fatal disease. No longer is this disease affecting only the population of our large metropolitan areas. It seems reasonable to believe that no community or even congregation of Christian believers will be spared the touch of some family involved either directly or indirectly. The need for supportive care will increase.

When Jesus sent out his twelve disciples, he told them among other things to "heal the sick." Physical healing may not be possible, but there is need for healing in broken relationships, broken spirits—that is, spiritual healing. The love message is all encompassing, far-reaching. Through it, God brings true life. Churches can become healing and teaching centers on responding with compassion.

Offer your services to hospice and support groups. There comes a time for family and friends, when all coping skills have been depleted and assistance is needed. Be there in their time of need. Don't be afraid to face death with them.

> The "poor," "dispossessed," and "outcast" for whom the prophets and Jesus had a special concern appear today as people with AIDS or ARC [AIDS-related complex] and, to a lesser degree, their loved ones and friends. For the church to ignore them and the varied needs that surround AIDS, to fail to respond and in the redemptive manner, and to abandon a people who have almost no one to cry out in their behalf for mercy and justice would constitute an abdication of its mission and a corruption of its identity. The church is challenged by AIDS to be the church. May it have the will, commitment, and courage to meet the challenge. By doing so, it will not only follow Jesus' example, but also set an example for others to follow.*

---

* Reprinted, with permission, from *AIDS: Personal Stories in Pastoral Perspective*, ed. Shelp, Sunderland, and Mansell, Page 200, copyright © 1986, The Pilgrim Press.

The Author

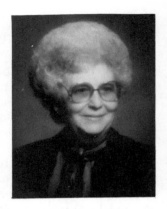

Helen M. Hostetler, the oldest of six children, was born to Oliver and Verna Bontrager near Middlebury, Indiana. The family lived on a truck farm where fruits and vegetables were grown to supplement their income. She came to know the joy that comes from inner peace and not outer security, a result of spiritual blessings and not material attainment. She is thankful that she grew up in a loving, secure Christian family.

After graduating from high school, she attended Goshen College at Goshen, Indiana, for a one-year pre-nursing program. She received her R.N. degree from the Mennonite Hospital School of Nursing in La Junta, Colorado.

For thirty-six years she lived with her husband, Marvin, and three children, Sheryl, Roger, and Janene, on their farm in McPherson County, Kansas. After they retired from farming and moved to McPherson in 1980, Marvin has been a salesman of real estate and insurance.

For thirty years Helen worked as a staff nurse and coordinator of education at the local hospital. For three years she was director of nursing service at the Cedars, an intermediate-care facility for 69 residents. Since then she has worked part-time for PORTAMEDIC doing medical exams for insurance applicants.

Through the years Helen has served in numerous positions for her church and conference. She teaches an adult Sunday school class and is active in prayer and Bible study groups.

Helen and her husband, Marvin, are members of the First Mennonite Church of McPherson, Kansas. They are sharing the story of their journey with AIDS with numerous groups and churches in the hope that care, love, and compassion might build bridges to overcome misunderstandings and broken relationships.

Their story is one of faith and courage in the face of stigma, fear, suffering, and loss.